Fearless Diet

Advance Praise for *Fearless Diet*

'*Fearless Diet* is a clinically relevant and behaviour-focused contribution to modern nutrition literature. Instead of prescribing restrictive meal plans, it adopts a coaching-based approach that mirrors real-world practice, teaching readers to interpret physiological feedback such as hunger, energy, sleep, cravings and digestion.

The book progresses systematically from mindset and behavioural awareness to applied nutrition, simplifying complex subjects like macronutrients, hydration and meal structuring without compromising scientific integrity. Its inclusive, non-fear-based philosophy supports sustainable metabolic health and long-term lifestyle change.

From a medical perspective, this work is a valuable educational tool for individuals navigating weight management and metabolic wellness. It reinforces a principle we emphasise in clinical care: lasting change begins with understanding the body, not controlling it.'

Dr Atul Sardana
Bariatric and Metabolic Surgeon,
Robotic and Laparoscopic Weight-Loss Specialist

'A practical guide taking you from food-fear-mongering to fitness-conquering. No more rigid rules, just the right tools.'

Dr SMiT
MBBS, CSCS

'*Fearless Diet* presents a practical, science-led approach to nutrition that focuses on understanding the body rather than following restrictive diets. Mitushi Ajmera's habit-based guidance simplifies complex concepts and promotes sustainable change. Clear, empowering, and grounded in real-world coaching, this book is a valuable resource for long-term health.'

Vikram Salwan
Director and CEO, QNT Sport India

'*Fearless Diet* is not about controlling food or the body; it is about understanding both. With rare clarity and compassion, Mitushi Ajmera replaces fear, guilt and confusion with awareness and sustainable habits. This is not a diet book; it is a lifelong framework for eating well and living better.'

Dr Sanjay Dhawan
CEO and Director, Medical Services,
Indira Gandhi Eye Hospital and Research Center

FEARLESS DIET

A Step-by-Step Guide to Balanced Nutrition

Mitushi Ajmera

BLOOMSBURY
NEW DELHI • LONDON • OXFORD • NEW YORK • SYDNEY

BLOOMSBURY INDIA
Bloomsbury Publishing India Pvt. Ltd
Second Floor, LSC Building No. 4, DDA Complex, Pocket C – 6 & 7,
Vasant Kunj, New Delhi, 110070

BLOOMSBURY, BLOOMSBURY INDIA and the Diana logo are trademarks of
Bloomsbury Publishing Plc

First published in India 2026

ISBN: PB: 978-93-69520-21-3; eBook: 978-93-69521-77-7

2 4 6 8 10 9 7 5 3 1

Typeset in Bembo by Manipal Technologies Limited
Printed and bound in India by Gopsons Papers Pvt. Ltd., Noida

To those who shaped my strength, and to those who are striving to build their own.

Contents

Foreword

I have never met Mitushi Ajmera in person. Yet, in many ways, I feel I know her. I know her thinking. I know her approach to diet, nutrition, lifestyle and exercise. And in today's noisy health ecosystem, that clarity of thought feels like a breath of fresh air.

I first came across her work on Instagram, a space unfortunately crowded with fake remedies, miracle claims and quick shortcuts to health. Amid all this noise, her voice stood out. She was not selling fear. She was not promising overnight transformation. Instead, she was advocating something far more powerful: a mindset and lifestyle change grounded in science, shaped by experience and driven by long-term well-being.

As a clinician, I see the consequences of health misinformation every single day. Patients and families often walk into my clinic carrying not just medical reports but also a heavy burden of confusion, fear and half-truths picked up from social media and well-meaning acquaintances. They are unsure whom to trust. They are anxious about eating the 'wrong' food, terrified of making 'mistakes', and constantly worried that one wrong choice might undo their recovery or harm their future. In this climate of uncertainty, balanced, evidence-based guidance is not just helpful; it is essential.

What sets *Fearless Diet* apart is that it does not attempt to control the reader's plate; it empowers the reader's mind. This is not a book of rigid meal plans, calorie charts or unrealistic templates. It is a thoughtfully designed coaching journey that teaches readers how to listen to their own bodies, understand feedback signals and make informed decisions in real-life situations. Through simple exercises, relatable examples and habit-based progression, Mitushi Ajmera helps readers build a practical framework that fits into Indian homes, busy work schedules, festivals, travel and social life. She does not create dependence on a system; she builds independence through understanding.

I believe this book has the potential to create a quiet but powerful shift in how individuals and families think about health. When people stop fearing food and start understanding it, they become more consistent, more confident and more resilient. Over time, this translates into better energy, better metabolic health, improved recovery and a stronger foundation for disease prevention. In my own field, I have seen how lifestyle choices influence outcomes, healing and quality of life. A book like *Fearless Diet*, when read and practiced sincerely, can help reduce avoidable suffering, prevent repeated cycles of weight loss and regain, and nurture a healthier relationship with the body across generations.

If you are holding this book in your hands, it already tells me something important about you. It tells me that you care about your health—that you are willing to learn, that you are open to change. You do not need perfection to move forward. You do not need extreme discipline or expensive foods. You do not need to transform overnight.

What you need is awareness, patience and consistency—and this book will help you build all three.

Read this book slowly. Practise what it teaches. Observe your body without judgement. Allow yourself the time to grow into healthier habits. There will be days when you follow everything perfectly, and days when you do not. Both are part of the journey. Progress is not measured by one meal, one week or one setback; it is measured by the direction in which you are moving over months and years.

It is my privilege to recommend *Fearless Diet* to you. Mitushi Ajmera has created a thoughtful, honest and scientifically grounded guide that respects both the complexity of the human body and the realities of daily life. This book does not promise miracles. It promises understanding—and that is far more valuable. I am confident that readers who engage with it sincerely will emerge not only better informed but also calmer, stronger and more empowered in their relationship with food and health.

I congratulate Mitushi Ajmera for this meaningful contribution to public health education and wish this book the wide readership it truly deserves.

Dr Jayesh Sharma
Cancer Surgeon,
ITSA Hospital, Raipur

Foreword

As I sit down to write this foreword, I am filled with excitement and anticipation.

Mitushi Ajmera's book on nutrition, *Fearless Diet*, is a breath of fresh air in an industry often dominated by fad diets and quick fixes. As a senior personal trainer, Pilates teacher and a nutritionist, with thousands of happy clients, Mitushi brings not just a wealth of knowledge and experience to the table but also an approach to nutrition that is both refreshing and empowering.

In this book, Mitushi shares her knowledge, tempered by her experiences with clients. She offers a holistic approach to nutrition that focuses on building healthy habits instead of following a specific diet. She suggests that readers ought to listen to the messages that the body continually sends. They will understand that lasting change comes from small, incremental steps and that every individual is unique.

One of the things that sets this book apart is its emphasis on positivity and self-care. Mitushi recognises that nutrition is not just about feeding our bodies in a highly regimented manner but also about understanding what the body wants. She offers practical tips and strategies for building healthy habits, managing stress and cultivating a positive body image.

Fearless Diet is a warm, supportive and non-judgemental offering from Mitushi, making readers feel like they are working with a trusted friend or mentor.

If you are looking for a book that will inspire and empower you to take control of your nutrition, look no further. This is a must-read for anyone seeking a healthier, happier relationship with food and their body. With its positive approach, practical tips and expert guidance, it is the perfect resource for anyone looking to make lasting changes and achieve optimal health and well-being.

Dilip Heble
Managing Director and CEO,
Gāyo Fitness Academy and Research Center
Private Limited

Letter to the Reader

Dear Reader, congratulations!

By being here, you have taken the first step: showing your intention and willingness to create change.

Whether your goal is to lose fat, feel more energetic, build sustainable eating habits or simply understand your body better, you are in the right place. This is not just a book to read; it is a book to use. You will not just read; you will practise as well. Each chapter will give you one practical action—small, realistic, and powerful—that you can start applying right away.

This book is not about forcing a new diet or striving for perfection. It is about providing you with the knowledge and confidence to nourish yourself with foods you enjoy and can access. My goal is simple: to help you become your own guide.

Before we begin, I want to explain why I believe that feeling amazing in your body has very little to do with a number on the scale and everything to do with understanding what helps you thrive.

My Journey—From Fads to Awareness

For the longest time, I believed that being thin automatically meant being healthy. Food was something to fill my stomach, not something I thought deeply about in terms of strength, energy, or recovery. Life, as it always does, had other plans to teach me.

After my first pregnancy, I naturally lost weight; not because I followed a plan but because life was busy. I did not understand nutrition then, but my body seemed to find its own rhythm.

Later, I stumbled into the world of fad diets. Someone told me about a 'magic diet' that promised fast results, and I believed them because I thought diets were good and were the only way to lose weight. I followed it diligently, and yes, the scale showed a quick drop. I was excited. I did not question whether what I was doing was sustainable or healthy. There was no social media then to verify information, and I was not even aware that something like poor-quality weight-loss methods existed.

My second pregnancy became the real turning point.

How It Started

After my second child was born, I reached my heaviest weight: 87 kg. I did not panic, but I understood it would take effort. I joined a gym and threw myself into exercise, believing that more sweat meant more success.

What My Exercise Used to Look Like

My workouts were driven by enthusiasm, not awareness. All I knew was that the more I sweat, the more I burn. I believed that intensity was everything. I often arrived late, skipped warm-ups, and stacked class after class—Zumba, body combat, circuit training—chasing fatigue rather than adaptation.

I was driven by excitement and the belief that 'more was better'. I felt proud seeing myself work hard each day.

Enthusiasm drove every rep, every set, every class.

What My Eating Used to Look Like

My breakfast at the time was straightforward and familiar:

- A glass of milk
- Two slices of toast with butter
- And my absolute favourite: *bhujia* sprinkled on top!

Yes, as a Marwari, *bhujia* felt comforting and cultural. Even when trainers suggested changes, I resisted: I could not imagine my morning without it. How could I give up something that brought me such joy?

I kept trying quick crash diets, thinking that was what my trainers meant.

My approach to food back then was also simple: 'Eat less.' I did not really know what 'less' actually meant or, more importantly, what 'better' could be.

And in the name of 'eating fewer calories', I would choose two salted crackers over a piece of fruit because the crackers had fewer calories and no sugar. I thought fewer calories and no sugar automatically meant a better choice.

The Wake-Up Call

Ironically, it was not the triumph but the collapse that followed immediately afterwards.

I lost 20–22 kg in about a year. On paper, it looked impressive. In reality, it was built on restriction, under-fuelling and relentless overtraining, with random diets and workouts stitched together by enthusiasm and misinformation. I hopped from one restrictive eating pattern to another, from one class to another, chasing the thrill of a smaller number on the weighing scale.

It worked...until my body gave out.

My body took the fall before my mind did.

Because I was dedicated to exercise, one of the trainers at my gym said, 'You exercise well. You are trainer material.' That single comment sparked a dream in me. It led me to sign up for my first Pilates workshop. I was not sure if I would be 'good enough', but I enrolled anyway, thinking it was more for my benefit than to become a teacher.

The irony deepened.

In the workshop, the teacher emphasised the calm philosophy of Pilates, which I ignored. Driven by the belief that if an exercise did not leave me shaking or burning, it was not effective, I practised excessively.

Within two weeks, my menstrual cycle arrived early, serving as my first signal that something was wrong. It was a clear sign that my body was responding to the deep internal work I was doing. I stopped briefly, but the damage had already begun.

The 'Payback' Time

Two days later, I woke up with a strange pain in my back. I brushed it off as a minor muscle twitch. I did what the old me did best—I pushed through, even going to the gym, hoping movement would make it disappear.

It did not lessen. It amplified.

By evening, I was bed-bound. The pain was electric; every step sent a pulse, like a surge of crushing current racing through my spine. When I finally saw a doctor, the diagnosis was clear: a grade 2 muscular injury caused by under-fuelling, overtraining and poor recovery.

Lying in bed with two young children depending on me, I was no longer thinking about fitness. I was afraid of being permanently broken.

But tragedy became my teacher. Lying in bed, wide awake and lost in thought, I kept asking one question over and over: *Why did this happen to me?*

The search for that answer led me into the world I now belong to—the fitness and nutrition industry. I devoured books with a hunger far greater than the diets I had starved myself on. I recovered with physiotherapy, and ironically, the same Pilates system I had over-practised became my key to healing when applied correctly.

The Shift

What I once used to punish my body became a means to rebuild it.

I learned that calories can be nutrient-dense or empty. That quality matters as much as quantity. That food is fuel, not something to earn or fear.

My downfall became my purpose.

What It Means Today

My mistake: Extreme workouts without optimal nourishment and recovery.

Fuelling my body with enough macronutrients, especially protein, never crossed my mind. Micronutrients like vitamin D, calcium, magnesium or even basic vitamin sufficiency were concepts I had not yet encountered.

Recovery was not part of my vocabulary. Post-workout food meant 'undoing' the work. Delayed nutrition signalled a job well done.

Looking back, it was not discipline; it was deprivation, stealthily disguised.

Science, nutrition and recovery were all the missing pieces in my story that was written on extremes.

This experience taught me something important: it is not only about the number of calories; it is also about the quality of nourishment, and in exercise, quality matters more than quantity.

I Turned the Tables

At forty-eight, I am a mother of two grown boys who chose to learn rather than give up. What began as personal struggle and self-experimentation led me to study, train and earn my place as a fitness trainer, Pilates and yoga teacher, fitness and sports nutritionist, and a senior master trainer. I am not someone who transformed overnight or figured everything out early. I am just an ordinary person who made mistakes, asked better questions, and turned lived experience into structured, science-backed guidance.

Today:

- I do not fear food, including *bhujia.*
- I do not exercise to tire myself out.
- I use science to maximise results with less effort.
- I fuel, recover and train with intention.

Feeling great is not about eating less and moving more; it is about eating better, training smarter, and taking care of the body you live in.

That is what I want to share with you.

This journey is not just about changing how you eat; it is about discovering how incredible you can feel when you approach your health with compassion instead of fear, love instead of deprivation, freedom instead of restriction, and curiosity instead of judgement. When you understand the science of nourishment, food stops being complicated and becomes joyful.

I have walked this path from confusion to clarity, from resenting my body to celebrating it. I have made mistakes that you can avoid, and now I am honoured to hand you the tools to make choices that will make you feel incredible every single day.

Thank you for trusting me to guide you on this journey. Use this book as your companion, write in it, highlight what resonates with you, and revisit it whenever you need encouragement. Take notes, experiment gently and, most importantly, be patient and kind with yourself. The most beautiful transformations do not happen overnight; they happen for those who stay consistent and kind to themselves.

Here is to a fitter, stronger, happier you!

With love and excitement for your journey,
Mitushi Ajmera

Introduction

Your Journey to a Fitter, Stronger, Happier You

You have already started your journey.

The moment you picked up this book, you chose to prioritise self-care.

This book is not just about weight loss; it is about becoming a better version of yourself, with weight loss being a bonus rather than an obsession.

The goal is not to wake up every day loving your body perfectly. Instead, the goal is to gently shift from restriction to nourishment, from criticism to respect.

When you take care of yourself, the number on the scale tends to take care of itself.

WHAT • HOW • WHY

'WHAT' Will We Do?

This book will guide you in reconnecting with the wisdom that resides within you. Most of us do not realise that we are constantly communicating with our bodies, even without speaking a single word. Every action we take—how we eat, move, rest, think, and even how we talk to ourselves—sends messages inward. Like any conversation, our bodies always respond. They communicate through energy, mood, cravings, sleep, cycles, aches and immunity. When we ignore these signals for too long, they manifest as symptoms.

The truth is: the body never stops communicating. The challenge lies not in hearing these messages but in understanding their language. We have been conditioned to override our bodies' signals: eating less, doing more, resting later, and pushing harder until we forget how to interpret what our bodies are trying to tell us. That is where we come together to help you reconnect.

'HOW' Will We Do?

One habit at a time.

The key to lasting transformation is not just willpower or motivation; it is about building habits.

Each chapter focuses on a single habit, giving you enough time for it to become established before introducing the next one. This approach helps prevent overwhelm and builds consistency.

'WHY' Will We Do?

Life can be unpredictable and challenging.

Many people find that tough days throw them off course.

This book provides a system designed to support you during those stressful times, not just when everything is going well.

This system is intended to work alongside your real life rather than against it.

Built on Three Pillars: Nourish, Move, Restore

Your journey to becoming fitter, stronger and happier rests on three interconnected pillars.

- **Nourish:** This pillar emphasises what you eat, how much you eat, and the consistency with which you nourish your body. Focus on choosing foods that provide energy, support metabolism, and help you feel satisfied and strong, without fear or restriction.

- **Move:** This pillar involves how you use your body. Movement is not about punishment or merely burning calories; it is about building strength, improving mobility, and enhancing resilience. The goal is to engage in activities that support your daily life, performance, and long-term health.
- **Restore:** Recovery is crucial. Adequate sleep, rest, and recovery allow your body to repair itself, regulate hormones, and adapt to both training and life stresses. Without proper restoration, neither nourishment nor movement can achieve their full benefits.

These pillars do not function in isolation.

When nourishment is adequate, movement becomes more effective.

When movement is appropriate, sleep improves.

When recovery is prioritised, the body responds better to both nutrition and exercise.

Sustainable health is achieved not by intensifying efforts in just one area but by supporting all three aspects together.

How to Use This Book

Use this book as your personal coach and let it guide you every day.

Read it. Write in it. Revisit it often.

Keep it on your kitchen counter rather than on your bookshelf.

This is a manual for living better, not a set of rules.

Getting Started on Your Journey

Take the time to read through each chapter and practise the habit it introduces before moving on to the next.

Give each habit the time it needs to become established before adding another.

Highlight the sections that resonate most with your life and goals. If necessary, set reminders or alarms to support you as you develop these new behaviours, but use them as encouragement rather than pressure.

Let us begin with Chapter 1 to understand how habits work and why they are more effective than relying on motivation alone.

1

Getting Started

'You do not rise to the level of your motivation, you fall to the level of your systems.'

—James Clear

What you do repeatedly and what you tell yourself consistently gradually shape your life.

Power of Habits

Consider this for a moment: What is the very first thing you do when you open your eyes? Chances are, you reach for your phone, you brush your teeth in the same order each time, brew your morning coffee in a set routine, sit on your preferred side of the bed, or use the same cup for your chai every day.

This chapter lays the foundation for how change actually works, through systems, not bursts of motivation.

These actions are not dramatic decisions made in the morning; they simply occur.

Why?

Because they are habits.

A habit is a tiny, repeated action that is quiet, automatic, and nearly invisible. You do not consciously decide to do it each time; you just do it. By the time you become aware of a habit, it has already taken control of your routine, operating efficiently without needing any permission.

Some habits are formed intentionally, while many develop accidentally.

Regardless, they shape your life.

The goal of this book is not to dismantle your entire life and rebuild it from scratch. Instead, it is to help you establish one essential habit first.

Take a Positive Approach

We will focus on incorporating positive actions rather than obsessively trying to eliminate 'bad' ones. By consistently adding nourishing behaviours, what no longer serves you will start to fade away on its own. Change does not occur through force; it happens through replacement.

Before we talk about food, fitness, or routines, we need to agree on the approach.

So, take a deep breath. There is no need to rush.

You have already taken a meaningful step by opening this book, which shows that you are ready for change. This process does not have to be frantic or forced; it simply requires preparation.

Acknowledge this progress and give yourself a pat on the back!

Remember to acknowledge every positive action you incorporate into your routine.

For example:

- That extra glass of water you drink? It matters. Give yourself a pat on the back.
- That walk you take during your calls? It counts. Give yourself a pat on the back.
- The fact that you are reading this to improve yourself? That is significant. Give yourself a pat on the back.

Do you see the secret that transforms everything?

You need to take positive actions to cultivate positive thoughts.

You cannot think your way to a healthier body, nor can you wish your way to more energy. However, you can definitely build your way there, one tiny positive action at a time, and appreciate each step you take. You do not need anyone else to motivate you; you can be your own motivator.

Understanding the Basics of Habits

Let me ask you again: When you wake up, do you consciously decide each step of your routine?

To change habits, you must first understand why the brain creates them.

Do you choose which hand to use while brushing your teeth?

Do you analyse how tightly to grip a spoon?

Of course not; you simply perform these actions.

These are not random occurrences; they are threads woven into the intricate web of habits that quietly govern your every move.

Imagine if you had to make a conscious choice for everything: when to breathe, how to walk, which hand to use, which foot moves first, the direction to turn the doorknob, and how tightly to grip a spoon. You would feel mentally exhausted before having breakfast!

So your brain performs a remarkable function: it automates familiar tasks, allowing you to conserve energy for more meaningful decisions.

If there were no habits?

Your brain constantly micromanages your movements, choices, and survival actions, which can lead to ongoing mental fatigue.

Habits Create Efficiency

Your brain strengthens actions that are repeated. When you practise certain actions often, they become faster, smoother, and require less mental effort over time.

Habits Create Autopilot Programming

Scientists estimate that 40–65 per cent of our daily actions are habits rather than conscious choices. Your brain does not evaluate whether a habit is 'good' or 'bad'; it simply makes repeated actions easier to perform.

Reaching for water at 6 a.m. or reaching for your phone at the same time gives the brain the same level of satisfaction. The brain seeks to minimise decision fatigue.

That is why one person may automatically grab fruit while another reaches for processed snacks. From the outside, it may appear as if one is exercising discipline, but it is really just a matter of different programming within the same habit system. The person who drinks eight glasses of water daily is not relying on motivation or willpower throughout the day; instead, staying hydrated has simply become a habit their brain has successfully adopted.

And that is the key truth: habits, not motivation, create lasting transformation.

Once you learn how your brain automates behaviour, you can re-train the system instead of fighting it. Transformation does not demand extraordinary effort when habits take control. The goal is to make healthy behaviours feel as effortless as brushing your teeth.

Why Habits Win Over Motivation

I have coached people for years and have noticed a recurring pattern.

The Motivation Pattern

People often start out highly motivated. They purchase gym memberships, stock their fridges with healthy food, and declare Monday as their day of transformation. For a while, everything appears perfect. However, life soon intervenes.

People do not go wrong because they lack effort but because they rely on the wrong tool.

The 'Life Happens' Phase

Work becomes chaotic. Children get sick. Deadlines loom. There are trips, festivals, celebrations, fatigue, and emotional stress. On good days, it is easy to eat a home-cooked meal, stay hydrated, and stay active.

But on difficult days, most people struggle to stay on track.

That is when the self-blame begins to kick in:

- 'I do not have the discipline.'
- 'I have lost my drive.'

But here is the truth: it was never solely about drive or motivation. Motivation can fluctuate when life gets chaotic. It is habits that keep you steady when things are not ideal.

The Real Test

Habits do not require debate.

- You drink water automatically.
- You feel hungry at predictable times.
- You move without negotiating with yourself.

You do not force yourself to navigate through chaos; instead, habits guide you through it.

The purpose of this book is to help you build something more substantial than a two-week reset: a lifelong framework you cannot easily undo. So, on your worst days, you will not think, 'I have to.' Instead, you will simply act.

How Habits Work in Your Body

Try this exercise to understand the power of habits.

Activity 1

Place this book down for a moment to do the exercise as you read along.

Ready?

You may sit comfortably in your chair or stand in a designated area.

First, fold your arms across your chest in the way that feels most natural to you. There are no specific instructions—just do it your way.

Done?

Take a moment to notice this position. Feel the weight of your arms. Notice the forearm that is on top. Is your right arm on top or your left? Notice the position of your wrist. Where are your fingers? Are they clenched in a fist, resting on your sleeves, or tucked under your arms? Notice how this feels in your shoulders and chest, and observe how both arms settle into a comfortable position.

Does this position not feel completely natural? There is no need for thinking or extra effort to adjust your fingers—it is as if your arms and fingers instinctively 'knew' where to go.

Now, unfold your arms.

Fold them again, but this time deliberately place the opposite arm on top.

Notice how this feels.

Does it feel strange or awkward? Perhaps a little uncomfortable? Does something feel 'off'? Do you find yourself wanting to switch back to your original position? Some people even describe this new way as feeling wrong.

The Science Behind What Just Happened

That discomfort you feel is your brain encountering a movement pattern it has not yet automated.

Over years of practice, your brain has developed a neural pathway that makes your usual arm crossing effortless. When you switch to a different pattern, you are asking your brain to attempt something new that has not yet been reinforced.

This process is how all habits are formed, from the way you walk to the things you reach for when you are stressed.

Change feels uncomfortable, not because it is wrong, but because it is unfamiliar.

That is why we will change habits gradually, one at a time, ensuring they become automatic before life puts them to the test.

Habits explain what we do automatically. Thoughts explain how those habits are born.

Now that you understand the power of habits, let us explore how your thoughts can accelerate this process.

The Power of Thoughts

If habits are the visible, automatic behaviours of your life, thoughts are the invisible roots that nourish and develop them. Every action, decision and behaviour begins as a conscious thought.

Initially, it is these conscious thoughts that form a habit, which your body and mind later perform without any conscious awareness.

The power of thought is not an abstract philosophical concept; it is a biological reality embedded in the very wiring of our brains.

How Thoughts Shape Your Brain Chemistry

When you consciously focus your thoughts and actions, you influence chemical messengers in your brain. For instance, thinking about hope, gratitude, or thankfulness can release dopamine and serotonin—neurotransmitters that promote feelings of motivation and well-being.

In contrast, constant worry, guilt and fear activate the brain's fear centre, triggering the 'fight or flight' response. This response floods your system with stress hormones like cortisol. When cortisol levels remain elevated, they suppress the activity of immune cells, making your body more vulnerable to infections. Over time, this biochemical environment determines not just your immune health but also your mood, resilience, and even creativity.[1]

Anecdote 1

COVID-19 and the role of awareness

Remember when COVID-19 first struck?

Fear was everywhere. People felt anxious and overwhelmed, constantly anticipating the worst. What stood out to me during that time, both personally and professionally, was how profoundly prolonged fear affected people's bodies.

As a coach, I had already observed how chronic stress alters appetite, sleep, recovery, and immunity. COVID-19 simply magnified this reality. Many people were not only grappling with a virus but also with months of heightened stress, poor sleep, irregular routines and emotional exhaustion.

Let me share my own experience during that period.

I was closely exposed to COVID-19.

I took precautions, stayed mindful, and focused on maintaining my routines as consistently as possible. I was not invincible, but I was resilient. Despite the uncertainty, I remained calm, regulated, and attentive rather than panicked.

The result?

I did not catch the virus.

Over the years, I have repeatedly observed a pattern that extends beyond just the COVID-19 pandemic.

Individuals who live in a constant state of fear and hyper-vigilance often experience more frequent illness, struggle to recover, and feel emotionally depleted.

In contrast, those who cultivate awareness, emotional regulation, and maintain steady routines tend to cope better with both physical and mental stressors.

This observation is not about denying reality or acting recklessly.

Rather, it is about recognising that fear itself creates a physiological state. When stress levels remain elevated for extended periods, the body stays in survival mode, redirecting energy away from repair, immunity, and recovery.

Awareness, calmness, and preparedness do not make anyone immune to challenges, but they do support the body's ability to respond effectively. I have witnessed this not only during the pandemic but also throughout my years of coaching people with diverse health backgrounds.

Fear can constrict the system, while awareness fosters resilience.

This lesson has stayed with me long after the pandemic has faded.

It is important to recognise that thoughts and actions are interconnected; they work together.

You cannot simply think your way into good health; you need to practise regularly.

The habits you create are the behavioural proof of the thoughts you put into action repeatedly, arising from a place of awareness.

Let me show you something amazing about the connection between your mind and body through a simple exercise.

Activity 2

The Mind–Body Connection

As you read, take your time to visualise what you see.

Ready?

You are holding a fresh, bright yellow lemon in your hand.

Feel its dimpled skin.

Notice its weight.

Imagine taking a sharp knife.

Now, with gentle strokes, cut the lemon in two.

Watch as the juice begins to drip from the fresh cut.

The citrus scent begins to fill the air.

Take one half of the lemon and place it between your teeth.

> Squeeze the juice from the lemon.
> Squeeze, squeeze, squeeze some more.
> Taste the sourness and that tanginess…
> Feel the zing as your teeth become sensitive.
> Now, pause.

What Just Happened?

Did your mouth water?

Perhaps you even scrunched up your face or felt your cheeks tighten.

That puckering reaction and the salivation are your body's responses in anticipation of food, even before you put it in your mouth—just from the mere thought of it.

Nothing physically happened; yet your body reacted.

This illustrates the power of the mind–body connection.

Your brain prepares your digestive system solely on the basis of imagination.

As you begin to think about and visualise that lemon, your brain sends a signal to your salivary glands, your stomach starts producing acid, and your entire digestive system prepares to receive a sour food.

Similarly, when positive thoughts are paired with repeated actions, they become automated. The brain learns to associate nourishment with safety, pleasure, and energy, rather than guilt and restriction.

This is why your mindset about food is just as important as what you choose to eat.

Do Positive to Become Positive

Why do I do what I do?

Most health strategies focus on restrictions: what you cannot eat, what you should avoid, and what you must steer clear of. This creates an attitude of negativity and limitation. Limitations lead to feelings of deprivation and resistance.

When you tell yourself 'I cannot have this', what happens?

Your attention becomes fixated on exactly that thing, every single time.

By concentrating on what you cannot have, you end up feeling deprived. Over time, this sense of deprivation can lead to rebellion.

You begin to dislike the food you eat.

You find yourself counting the days until your diet ends.

If something unexpected happens, you might quit and blame that event for throwing you off track.

We are going to take a different approach.

Let us focus on what you enjoy and what positive steps you should take.

Instead of saying, 'Do not eat this', I will encourage you to think about 'What can we add?'

Starting today, I want you to embrace the act of eating:

- Eat to nourish yourself.
- Eat to celebrate life.

By adopting this mindset, you will look forward to eating and enjoying without any desire to quit. In a world that often emphasises elimination diets and forbidden foods, a subtle change in attitude can lead to positive actions.

Instead of saying 'Do not eat cookies', we should focus on 'Let us add protein to your morning.'

Rather than saying 'Avoid sugar', we can explore the best times to enjoy it.

Instead of fearing deep-fried food, let us discover how good-quality fats and proper portion sizes can make you feel better.

When nourishing actions increase, what needs to be reduced will naturally fall away—without guilt or force.

We will not demonise any food—whether it is sugar, rice, your favourite sweets at festivals, or your pizza treats.

There are no forbidden foods; there are nourishing foods and soulful treats. There should be awareness and choice, not guilt and shame. This approach makes your diet inclusive rather than exclusive.

Biryani is not the enemy.

Chocolate is not hindering your progress.

The sweet lassi you enjoy on hot summer afternoons is not a setback.

These are your foods, your traditions, your festivals, your sources of happiness.

It is not about being perfect; it is about finding balance, being aware, and making conscious choices.

Baby Steps, Big Transformation

Sustainable change occurs in a manner similar to how skills are learned progressively.

> **Sustainable change is never dramatic; it is quiet, progressive and repeatable.**

Think of it like learning to play a musical instrument. First, you are taught how to hold the instrument correctly. Once that becomes second nature, you start with simple notes. Next, you progress to basic tunes, followed by more complex pieces. Each skill builds upon the previous one until you can play an entire musical sequence without having to consciously think about where to place your fingers or how to control your breath.

This is the approach taken by this book.

Each chapter introduces one habit to practise until you reach the end of the next chapter, where you add the next.

A Pause Is Not Failure; Quitting Is

Anecdote 2

Adversity turned into opportunity

Adversity can become an opportunity for growth and learning if we remain attentive to the lessons it offers.

For me, it began as an ordinary day. I was returning home after finishing my classes, only to discover that the elevators were out of service. My apartment was on the seventeenth floor, and staying downstairs was not an option, so I decided to take the stairs. It seemed daunting, as I had never climbed more than two floors at a time. But I started anyway.

I paused a few times to catch my breath, but I eventually made it to the top.

That one climb did not just take me home; it sparked an idea: 'What if I did this more often?'

I began climbing the stairs intentionally, incorporating it into my exercise routine twice a week. I progressed from seventeen floors to twenty, then forty, and eventually eighty. By the end of the month, I was climbing a hundred floors.

The practice greatly improved my confidence, strength, stamina, speed, and self-belief—far more than my comfort zone ever did. Now I climb 120 floors, or 2,400 steps, in under an hour as part of my workout.

The real surprise came when I impulsively enrolled in a vertical marathon and placed second in my category. This achievement was not because of any extraordinary feats but rather because I did not give up in the face of adversity.

Seeing my progress inspired my students to join in as well, transforming it into a fun activity for all of us. So remember: never quit, as you never know what new opportunities may arise.

Small actions can lead to significant outcomes, as long as you do not give up. Taking a pause is not a waste of time; it is an opportunity to reset your energy so you can push further.

This is similar to interval training, where effort is followed by rest and then repeated. That is how transformation occurs. Progress is rarely linear; it tends to zigzag.

Here are a couple of examples of how small actions can add up:

- Eating one extra serving of vegetables each day results in 365 nutrient-rich servings a year.
- Taking a 10-minute walk after dinner adds up to 5 hours of movement in a month.

Remember, this journey is not a race, and you are not competing against anyone else.

It is about you leading yourself, cheering yourself on, rewarding yourself, and giving yourself a pat on the back.

As I always say, health and fitness cannot be outsourced; you are the sole proprietor.

If it is about you, then it is truly you versus yourself. So, do not rush.

Rushing prevents habits from settling in. If you struggle to complete a certain task, that is okay—give yourself more time. What matters is that you keep moving forward. You are constantly learning, and your brain is making connections that will ultimately take you where you want to be.

Did you miss a day? Reset tomorrow.

Did you slip up? Learn from it.

Instead of feeling guilty, ask yourself: What can I do to make it work next time?

Prepare a Plan B before tough days arrive. This is constructive problem-solving rather than feeling helpless and guilty.

You are not becoming someone new; you are evolving into a healthier version of yourself.

Myths and Truths

1. *Myth:* 'Habits take 21 days to form.'
   Truth: This widely held belief is scientifically wrong. Research[2] shows that forming habits can take anywhere from 18 to 254 days, depending on factors such as the complexity of the behaviour, the environment, and the emotional connection to it. Ultimately, it is consistency—not a specific timeframe—that truly helps establish habits.
2. *Myth:* 'Fear is just an emotion; it does not affect the body.'
   Truth: Fear activates the stress response, lowers immunity, tightens muscles, affects digestion, and weakens clarity. Your thoughts directly influence physiology.
3. *Myth:* 'Motivation or willpower builds habits.'
   Truth: Motivation and willpower are unreliable; they can fluctuate and are often mood-dependent. Instead, effective systems, routines, tracking, and a conducive environment are key to building habits. While motivation or willpower may start the process, it is structure that helps habits endure.
4. *Myth:* 'If I miss one day, my habit is broken.'
   Truth: Missing a day does not significantly affect long-term habit formation. You can always restart a habit, and you can repeat this process as many times as necessary whenever you feel it has been disrupted.

5. *Myth:* 'I need to change everything at once.'
   Truth: Real change occurs through tiny adjustments rather than dramatic overhauls. Small, sustainable habits accumulate over months and years; that is where true transformation happens.
6. *Myth:* 'Positive thinking alone is enough.'
   Truth: While thoughts shape intentions, actions lead to results. Relying solely on positive thinking without positive behaviour or action can become a form of escapism. True transformation occurs when thought is paired with consistent habits.
7. *Myth:* 'Thoughts are harmless.'
   Truth: Thoughts shape neural pathways, emotional responses, decision-making, and identity. Repeated thoughts, whether positive or negative, develop into automatic patterns that influence behaviour.

To Reiterate

- Brain automates repetition; it does not judge good or bad.
- Habits beat willpower on tough days.
- Change is built brick by brick, not overnight.
- Fear and guilt 'out'; awareness and conviction 'in'.
- Positivity starts from doing, not wishing.
- Pause → Reset → Move → Repeat.
- Awareness + positive actions = sustainable transformation.
- Transformation never moves in a straight line; it goes zigzag.

A Note from Me to You

I have guided thousands of people through this journey, and I have witnessed the magic that unfolds when we approach change with love instead of fear, with addition instead of avoidance, with freedom instead of restriction, and with patience instead of urgency. When we stop labelling foods as 'good', 'bad', or 'miraculous', we reclaim our power to eat with awareness rather than fear. You already possess everything you need within you. This book is simply here to help you unlock that potential.

Habit 1

Your first habit to practise: 'Smile more'

Now that you understand how your actions fuel your thoughts, let us apply this to building positive habits.

Starting today, I encourage you to carry a smile when entering an elevator, using an escalator, going to the gym, shopping at the grocery store, or arriving at your office. This is not about forced positivity or pretending everything is perfect. It is about understanding that positive emotions start with you and create a ripple effect that benefits everyone around you.

Here is what happens when you smile at a stranger: they almost always smile back. It is an automatic human response. Think about it—when someone enters an elevator and genuinely smiles at you, you find yourself smiling back, even if you do not know them. In that moment, you have created something powerful. You have initiated a positive interaction that lifts both of you.

What is the outcome of this interaction?

This simple exchange triggers the release of feel-good hormones in your brain. When you smile, your brain again releases endorphins, serotonin, and dopamine—the natural chemicals that reduce stress and create feelings of happiness. The person receiving your smile experiences the same chemical boost. You have literally made yourselves both healthier with a single facial expression.

This practice trains your mind to seek out positive interactions instead of focusing on what is wrong. As you cultivate more positive emotions throughout your day, negative feelings and stress naturally begin to diminish. You are creating an internal environment of happiness and calm, which directly impacts your physical health. Your stress hormones decrease, your immune system strengthens, and your overall well-being improves—all without making any dietary changes yet.

Remember, you have the ability to lift someone's spirits. Perhaps that person in the elevator was having a tough morning, and your smile was just what they needed. Even though you will never fully know the effect of this simple act, you will definitely notice its positive effects on your own mood and energy throughout the day.

2

Set Your Baseline

NOW THAT YOU COMPREHEND the significance of habits and how this journey will progress, it is time to establish your baseline.

Understanding Your Starting Point

Every transformation, whether in health, fitness, or life, needs a starting point. This baseline is not for judgement or attaching personal worth to a number; it serves as the foundation for tracking progress, observing changes, and celebrating growth over time.

We begin by gathering your basic information: current weight, body measurements, and, in some cases, photographs or fitness performance markers. This may seem intimidating, but remember, these are not judgements about you; they are simply data points that will help you assess your progress.

A baseline is not a judgement. It is a reference.

Why Measure Progress?

'What gets measured, gets managed.'

—Peter Drucker

It is easy to dismiss numbers and think, 'I will just go by how I feel.' While how you feel is important, objective measurements provide us with clear evidence of our progress. But it is essential to understand this: numbers do not define you; they simply inform you.

You cannot change what you do not first observe.

Measurements are checkpoints.

They help you understand where you started and where you are headed. They help connect the dots between your actions and their outcomes.

When you review these numbers weekly or monthly, you will start to notice trends.

For instance, your weight might remain the same while your waistline has decreased. Alternatively, maybe you have dropped 2 kg, but your waist measurements have not shifted yet. Each of these changes tells us something unique about what is happening in your body.

This practice is not about achieving excessive happiness, feeling shame or guilt, or comparing ourselves to others. Instead, it focuses on acknowledgement, responsibility, observation and learning. And, equally important, it is about celebrating progress, even the small steps. If things do not change, you will have all the information needed to trace back to where things might have gone off track.

Feelings are valuable. Data gives direction.

Consider this: you may have attended a party or just returned from a holiday. The next morning, you still weigh yourself and take your measurements.

> **Weight tells you how heavy you are. Measurements tell you what changed.**

Why?

Not to beat yourself up, but to understand how different foods, alcohol, sleep, and activity levels affect your body. This awareness helps you to learn, adjust, and move forward more mindfully.

The Scale Versus the Tape

Why does girth matter more?

Most people are conditioned to believe that weight is the ultimate indicator of progress. However, relying solely on weight can be quite misleading.

Here is why:

- Muscle and fat have very different densities. Imagine holding 1 kg of iron versus 1 kg of cotton; both weigh the same, but iron is compact and dense, while cotton is fluffy and takes up much more space. Similarly, 1 kg of muscle is dense, tight, and compact, whereas 1 kg of fat is bulkier and takes up more space. This means it is possible to lose fat while gaining muscle simultaneously. On the scale, the number might not budge significantly, but when you look in the mirror, you might notice that your body appears leaner and more defined, and your clothes fit better. That is real progress, even if the scale does not reflect it.
- Girth measurements reveal the real story. When fat is lost from your waist, hips, chest, or thighs, the tape measure will show reductions—even if your weight

on the scale stays the same. This is the transformation you can genuinely feel and see in your daily life.

- Water weight and muscle loss can skew our understanding of progress. Sometimes you might notice the scale dropping by 2–3 kg quickly, but if your measurements have not changed, that weight loss is likely water or muscle loss rather than fat loss. This is not the kind of progress we want.

Fat and muscle weigh the same, but they do not behave the same.

This is why we track both weight and measurements; using one without the other does not provide a complete picture.

Anecdote 3

The weight that did not move, but everything else did

Once, a twenty-eight-year-old woman from Raipur enrolled in my nutrition and exercise coaching programme. She was meticulous, weighing herself every day, logging her meals honestly, and updating me through the week. She followed every instruction, took weekly measurements, and fully engaged in the process.

But by the end of Week 3, she had not sent me her measurements. When I asked why, she replied, disappointed, 'Ma'am, there is no change. My weight has not moved.'

I insisted she check anyway.

When the results came in, I was stunned.

She had lost 6 inches from her waist in just 21 days.

I called her immediately.

'What are you even saying? Is 6 inches gone, not progress?'

She hesitated and replied, 'But ma'am, my weight is the same. I have not lost anything.'

So I asked her how she felt.

Her hunger was better, her sugar cravings had settled, her energy was good, and her clothes were looser.

I clarified what was really going on: 'You have likely gained some muscle, improved your bone density, and your muscles are storing more glycogen and therefore more water. All of this adds weight. Fat, on the other hand, is like cotton: light, fluffy, and bulky. Lean mass is like iron: compact and heavy. You lost fat but gained strength.'

With this understanding of the science, her disappointment transformed into motivation.

The Right Pace of Progress

When you understand the science, disappointment turns into motivation.

Fast loss is seductive; sustainable loss is powerful.

A common mistake people make is chasing rapid weight loss. It is tempting to seek big numbers quickly, but extreme calorie deficits often backfire. They can cause you to lose not only fat but also muscle, slow your metabolism, and make the weight-loss process unsustainable.

Instead, focus on achieving a gradual, steady loss of fat while preserving muscle.

Losing 2 kg of pure fat per month is considered an athletic rate of weight loss.

While 1 kg of fat loss per month may seem slow, it adds up to 12 kg of pure fat loss in a year. That is significant progress, especially when it is muscle-preserving, sustainable, and geared towards the long term.

Here is a helpful reference point:

On average, every 1 kg of fat loss should show at least 1 inch of reduction in body measurements. Some of my clients have even lost 3–6 inches from their waists with just 1 kg of weight loss. This clearly shows that the scale does not tell the entire story.

Why Muscle Preservation Is Non-Negotiable

> **Weight loss without muscle preservation is a short-term win and a long-term loss.**

Our aim is not only to lose fat but also to preserve and ideally build muscle.

Why?

Muscle is a metabolically active tissue that burns calories even when at rest. It helps maintain a healthy hormone balance and keeps your body strong and functional. The more muscle you have, the higher your metabolism will be, which makes it easier to maintain fat loss.

On the other hand, losing muscle makes it more difficult to lose fat in the future. This is why crash diets and extreme calorie restrictions often fail: while people may lose weight, a significant portion of it comes from muscle and water. This leaves them feeling weaker, less energetic, and more prone to regaining weight.

Therefore, our progress markers should always focus on fat loss and muscle retention. This combination is the key to achieving sustainable results.

Change the Way You See Progress

Think about the last time someone complimented you.

> **No one compliments a number. They compliment how you look.**

Did they start by asking about your weight?

Or did they simple say, 'You look great!'

No one cares about the number on the scale. People notice your posture, your glow, your energy, how your clothes fit, and how confident you appear. All of this is a result of fat loss, muscle preservation and improved health, not from fixating on a specific number.

This is why I always remind my clients: the scale does not give the complete picture, but the mirror and your clothes do.

What to Remember Before We Begin

- Measurements are tools, not judgements. They help us observe trends and adjust our strategies.
- Weight is only one part of the picture. Girth measurements are often more reliable in reflecting true changes in body composition.
- Muscle and fat behave differently. You can appear leaner and fitter even if the scale does not move much.
- Sustainable fat loss is a gradual process. Losing 1–2 kg of fat per month is a realistic and healthy goal.
- It is important to preserve muscle. It supports metabolism, functionality, and long-term results.
- Your worth is not measured in numbers. Progress is about how you feel, how you move, and the confidence you carry.

The Mindset to Carry Forward

The journey of transformation is not just about reaching a specific weight; it is about becoming a stronger, healthier, and more confident version of yourself. While the scale provides information, it does not define who you are. True progress comes from a combination of fat loss, muscle preservation, improved health markers, and feeling good in your own skin. Most importantly, you have the power to shape your body, because your body is your business, not anyone else's.

Progress is a pattern, not a daily result.

So the next time you step on the scale or take a measurement, do not think of it as a judgement. Instead, it is feedback—just a small piece of the larger picture that helps guide you towards lasting change. So let us get started!

Taking Your Measurements

For accurate measurements, take them first thing in the morning, ideally in light clothing, before eating or drinking anything other than water.

Your body is not a project to fix; it is a system to understand.

Today's date: __________ **Weight:** __________

Please take the following measurements using a measuring tape (in inches or cm):

Body Part	Measurement	Body Part	Measurement
Neck	________	Shoulder	________
Chest	________	Biceps	________
Waist (narrowest part)	________	Waist (belly button)	________
Waist (2 inches below belly button)	________	Hips	________
Thigh	________	Calf	________

Table 2.1: *Recommended body measurement points for tracking changes in body composition over time*

Why These Specific Measurements Matter?

Your waist measurement is one of the most reliable indicators of internal health, as it reflects changes in visceral fat surrounding your organs and any bloating. This area is where we typically store the most fat, so we measure it at three points.

In men, tracking the three waist measurements weekly is usually sufficient, while additional measurements can be taken monthly.

In women, it is important to note that the chest is also an area where fat is stored, as breasts are primarily made of fat tissue. Therefore, women should take at least these four measurements—waist and chest—weekly, while other measurements can be taken monthly.

The measurements of your biceps, hips and thighs may not provide a clear picture on their own, as these areas are also where we build thick muscles. Therefore, a gain or loss in these measurements can give misleading signals when considered individually. When evaluated together, they provide a more accurate picture of your body composition changes than the scale alone can.

Where fat leaves first is not random; it is biological.

Your Food Awareness Log

Based on my coaching experience, individuals who maintain their logs for at least three to six months tend to make the most progress. This is not because logging itself creates change but because it fosters self-awareness.

When you write things down, you become your own evaluator, prompting you to think more constructively. For example, you may think, 'I could have eaten that instead of this', or you may begin searching for healthier food alternatives in this book to make better choices in the future. Gradually, you start making these decisions without needing anyone else to point out where you could improve. This gentle awareness ultimately leads to better choices.

Begin by logging your meals for today. If you can, also record what you ate yesterday. Aim to record your meals for at least three days, so you can compare your entries 'at the start' of the book with those at the 'end of the book' to observe your progress and celebrate any changes.

After these three days, create a separate diary for regularly tracking your food intake.

Awareness creates change long before discipline does.

Day 1

- **Date:** ________________
- **Wake-up time:** ________________
- **Sleep time:** ________________
- **Observations/notes:** ________________________

Time of the Meal	Food Item	Quantity	Ingredient Details

Table 2.2: *Daily meal and habit tracker to record wake-up time, sleep time, food intake, quantities and ingredients*

Day 2

- **Date:** _______________
- **Wake-up time:** _______________
- **Sleep time:** _______________
- **Observations/notes:** ______________________

Time of the Meal	Food Item	Quantity	Ingredient Details

Table 2.3: *Daily meal and habit tracker to record wake-up time, sleep time, food intake, quantities and ingredients*

Day 3

- **Date: ________________**
- **Wake-up time: ________________**
- **Sleep time: ________________**
- **Observations/notes: ________________________**

Time of the Meal	Food Item	Quantity	Ingredient Details

Table 2.4: *Daily meal and habit tracker to record wake-up time, sleep time, food intake, quantities and ingredients*

How To Track Progress

Progress involves much more than just the numbers you see on a scale or a measuring tape. True transformation is reflected in how you feel, how well you sleep, and how your body functions each day. That is why I encourage you to track these important indicators along with your measurements.

Start observing the following to gain a comprehensive understanding of your progress, and make sure to note these in the observations section of every food log.

> **A healthier body behaves differently, not just weighs less.**

Daily measurements

- Water intake: ______ litres per day
- Sleep duration: ________ hours per day
- Sleep quality: Poor/Good/Excellent
- Energy levels throughout the day: Poor/Good/Excellent

Weekly assessments

- Sugar cravings: High/Moderate/None
- Hunger pangs/craving for snacks: Often/Moderate/Rarely
- Bowel movement: Regular/Constipation/Frequent indigestion
- Flatulence/gas/acidity/heartburn: Severe/Moderate/Rarely

Why These Matter

These indicators show how effectively your body is responding to the changes you are making. When you begin to nourish yourself properly and build healthy habits, you will notice improvements in several areas.

Better hydration can lead to increased energy levels and reduced sugar cravings. Quality sleep helps regulate hunger. Regular bowel movements indicate that your gut health is improving. Finally, stable energy throughout the day suggests that your blood sugar is becoming more balanced.

Most people notice improvements in hunger pangs, sugar cravings, and energy levels within the first week. By the second week, digestion begins to improve. By the third week, cravings significantly decrease.

Better nourishment shows up in sleep, energy, and digestion before it shows on the scale.

Take 10 minutes each week to review your progress in these areas and look for patterns.

Setting Your Intentions

What to Expect from This Journey

This is real-life health, not textbook perfection.

Based on Chapter 1, we will delve into practical steps you can start implementing right away. This is not idealistic health information that looks good only on paper but is impractical for everyday kitchens, busy schedules and real families. Each chapter will build upon the previous one, creating a comprehensive system for lifelong health that can be tailored to your unique situation.

You can expect a gradual transformation; there are no overnight miracles. Remember, progress does not follow a straight line; it often moves in a zigzag pattern. So, do not get overly excited with every weight loss or too discouraged with every weight gain.

Regular weekly measurements will help you stay on track with your goals. At the end of each month, review the numbers to understand the overall impact and compare the results quarterly to maintain motivation and prepare for the next quarter.

Additionally, remember that small, daily good deeds contribute to your overall health and vitality, helping you thrive in the long term.

One Commitment I Want You to Make to Yourself

Treat yourself with the same kindness that you would show a small baby. When introducing a new food, do so gradually and in smaller quantities.

Consider this: when a baby refuses to eat, you gently and tactfully try to feed them, which could also mean altering the recipe or making the food more appealing. Similarly, I do not want you to force yourself to eat anything that you do not like. Instead, I will explain why certain foods might be beneficial and how you can gradually incorporate them into your routine if they are important to your health. This may require altering the recipe.

You should pursue this when you are somewhat convinced and are willing to try, because the body responds more effectively when the mind is in alignment.

> **Progress happens faster when the body feels safe; it shows up on the scale.**

This is not about striving for perfection or avoiding mistakes entirely. Rather, it is a promise to treat yourself with kindness and to trust the process, even when you do not see immediate, measurable results.

Anecdote 4

The client who lost on weekdays and 'gained' on weekends

One of my clients had a distinct pattern in her progress. Every Monday, she would send me her weight and measurements, and each time, she sounded defeated.

'I do not know why this keeps happening,' she would say. 'I eat well and follow the plan, but I always gain weight over the weekends.'

To help her understand what was happening, I suggested an experiment: for four weeks, we would record her measurements twice a week—once on Friday and again on Monday.

A noticeable pattern emerged: from Monday to Friday, she typically experienced weight loss. From Friday to Monday, she would either gain a little weight or retain water, even though she was not overeating or exceeding her calorie deficit.

Every Monday, it felt as if she were back to square one.

But at the end of the month, I shared some surprising news: Despite the fluctuations, she had lost 2 inches around her belly over the four weeks. Her fat loss graph was not a straight line; instead, it resembled a zigzag pattern that still trended downward.

Why was she gaining weight on weekends despite eating well?

Her weekend routine was different, which affected how her body functioned, even when her calorie intake was controlled.

She engaged in more intense physical activities on weekends. This increased activity led to muscle inflammation, more microtears, greater glycogen storage, and increased water retention. As a result, her weight and waist circumference temporarily increased.

Even slight changes in salt intake, electrolyte levels, and water consumption can lead to quick shifts in water retention. Additionally, her sleep schedule was disrupted; staying up late and altering her circadian rhythm increased cortisol levels, contributing to water retention.

Despite her efforts being on track, her body's recovery responses made her weekend measurements look less favourable.

When I showed her the trend for the entire month, which showed a steady downward slope despite the weekly fluctuations, she began to understand that progress is rarely linear. It is often a messy, zigzagging path that still moves forward. Once she realised this, she stopped fearing Mondays.

Myths and Truths

1. *Myth:* 'If the scale is not moving, I am not progressing.'
   Truth: Fat loss and weight loss are not the same.
   You can lose fat and gain muscle simultaneously. This means your weight remains the same, even as your body becomes leaner, firmer, and healthier.
2. *Myth:* 'The measuring tape does not fluctuate.'
   Truth: It does. Water retention, inflammation, menstrual cycle, sodium intake, and heavy training days can all temporarily increase measurements.
   However, unlike weight, tape measurements better reflect the true direction of change over time.

Zigzag progress is still progress.

3. *Myth:* 'Muscle gain makes you look bulky.'
   Truth: Muscle is your metabolic gold. It shapes your body, tightens your frame, protects your joints, improves insulin sensitivity, preserves bone density and promotes healthy ageing. When combined with fat loss, muscle gain can actually make your body look leaner rather than bulkier. It is the fat covering the muscles that creates a bulky appearance. By further reducing fat, you can achieve a leaner look.

4. *Myth:* 'My body should make progress daily.'

   Truth: Progress should be observed as trends or patterns over time rather than on a daily basis. Your body is affected by various factors, including sleep, stress, sodium intake, recovery, hormones, training intensity, and even the weather. Daily fluctuations are insignificant; instead, it is the weekly and monthly patterns that truly matter.

5. *Myth:* 'If weight goes up overnight, I must have done something wrong.'

   Truth: Overnight weight gain is typically due to factors such as water retention, glycogen storage, inflammation from training, or delays in digestion rather than fat gain. To actually gain fat, a consistent calorie surplus over several days is needed.

6. *Myth:* 'The weighing scale is useless.'

   Some nutritionists say this with good intentions, but it can be misleading.

   Truth: You do not need to throw the scale away; you just need to stop placing so much emphasis on it. The scale provides one piece of data, but it does not tell the whole story. Use it as a tool to track trends over weeks rather than as a judgement of your self-worth.

7. *Myth:* 'Weight loss should be linear if you are doing everything right.'

   Truth: Body transformation is always a zigzag. Daily numbers lie. Weekly numbers confuse. Monthly numbers tell the real story.

To Reiterate

- Self-awareness is your starting point; by recording your details, you have begun the journey of taking the onus of your health onto yourself.
- Habits trump motivation every time; lasting change comes from building automatic behaviours, not relying on motivation that comes and goes.
- Positive actions create positive outcomes; you cannot think your way to health; you have to take positive steps to become positive.
- Addition beats restriction; when you focus on what to add to your life, what is not serving you naturally gets crowded out without a fight.
- Weight loss is just a bonus; your real goal is becoming fitter, stronger, and happier. The scale will follow when you take care of yourself.
- Measurements track progress, not worth; your baseline numbers are a starting point for celebration, not judgement. They show how far you have come, not how far you have to go.
- Your brain does not distinguish between good and bad habits; it just automates whatever you repeat. This is your secret weapon for transformation.
- Baby steps lead to big changes; small, consistent actions compound over time to create remarkable results.
- You are the sole proprietor of your health; it is you for you, you versus you. Take ownership because you are the only one who can create this change.
- Kindness and patience are non-negotiable; treat yourself like you would treat a small child learning something new. Be truthful to yourself and let you help you.

A Note from Me to You

Measuring is not an obsession; it is clarity. The scale alone cannot tell you whether you are losing fat, preserving muscle, or simply shifting water; that is why I talk about looking beyond one number. Muscle is your metabolic asset, your armour for ageing, hormones, and long-term health, and preserving it must always be a priority. Food logs and simple tracking tools are not meant to restrict you; they help you see patterns you would otherwise miss, so you can adjust with confidence instead of guessing. Progress is not just how much you weigh; it is how you feel, move, and recover. When you measure the right things, you manage the right things.

Habit 2

Finding 'good' in others

Now that you have the starting measurements and understand how powerful your thoughts are in creating physical responses, let us apply this to adding to our positive habits.

Starting today, I want you to practise a simple but transformative exercise: genuinely try to find at least one good thing in every person you encounter. This could be anything—the way someone holds the door, their choice of clothing, how patient they are with their child, their smile, or even something as simple as appreciating that they said 'thank you'.

The key is to actively look for something positive rather than focusing on what might be wrong or annoying.

When possible, let them know. People love hearing good things about themselves. A simple 'I love the way you are carrying this outfit' or 'Thank you for being so patient' can brighten someone's entire day.

This practice trains your brain to seek out positivity rather than problems. When you make it a habit to look for what is good, your mind automatically starts scanning for positive things everywhere, including in yourself and your own choices.

This shift in mental focus has direct physical benefits, as we learned earlier. When your brain is focused on these positive experiences, it will increase feel-good chemicals—serotonin and dopamine, which will in turn reduce stress hormones like cortisol as they are inversely proportional. That is the natural way of balancing these hormones; controlled stress hormones mean better metabolism, improved immune function, and more stable energy throughout the day.

As you practise finding 'good' in others, you start patting your back for making the efforts and doing the tasks that this book recommends. This will start to translate into a better relationship with yourself, making you more compassionate with yourself. You will naturally start finding good in yourself and your health choices, too. The shift from criticising yourself for not being perfect to noticing and appreciating the positive steps you are taking will set off a cascade of positivity. This will create a cycle of encouragement and enjoyment that will make healthy habits much easier to incorporate and maintain.

Most frustration comes from misunderstanding how the body actually works.

3

The Basics of Good Nutrition

> **Nutrition should support life, not dominate it.**

NUTRITION IS ONE OF the most important pillars of health.

Good nutrition is built on balance, variety, and quality.

It involves obtaining the right mix of nutrients in amounts that meet your body's specific needs. There is no one-size-fits-all solution, as each individual has unique requirements based on factors such as age, activity level, health status, goals, and professional or personal limitations. At its core, good nutrition emphasises whole, natural, and minimally processed foods that provide the body with steady energy and resilience. Proper nutrition supports the gut microbiome, regulates hormones, reduces inflammation, and strengthens the immune system.

What, when and how we eat significantly influences how we feel throughout the day. Practising mindful eating and paying attention to our hunger and fullness cues helps us connect with our body's internal signals.

A sound approach to nutrition should feel sustainable and adaptable to your lifestyle rather than restrictive or temporary. Ultimately, it is not about achieving perfection or adhering to strict food rules, but about consistently making choices that enhance the body's function today while also protecting long-term well-being.

If it is not sustainable, it is not healthy, no matter how 'clean' it looks.

The Truth About What Nutrition Cannot Do

While nutrition is important, it is often misunderstood as a magic solution. Making good food choices can have a significant impact, but there are limits to what nutrition or any single food can achieve.

There is no superfood. Instead, there are well-used foods and those that are overhyped.

No single food is cure-all.

The term 'superfood' has no scientific or regulatory definition and is largely a marketing label, often used to shape consumer perception rather than reflect a formal nutritional category. The term is mostly used to promote certain foods by exaggerating their benefits. When a food seems too promising or is marketed as a singular solution, it usually ignores an essential truth: the body requires a variety of nutrients from different foods to function optimally. Good health is built on a combination of foods and consistent eating habits, not on relying on a single standout ingredient.

In the European Union, foods cannot be marketed with implied health superiority, such as being labelled as a 'superfood', unless they are supported by authorised health claims backed by scientific evidence.[1]

So, remember: there is no perfect food or diet that can magically change or cure a person overnight. In reality, actual good nutrition requires many foods that work collectively and slowly.

Health is built through patterns, not products.

The body takes time to adapt, and only then does it begin to show changes with the new way of eating. Hence, change requires consistency over time. Subtle changes may be observed within days, while more significant changes may take weeks or months, depending on the severity of the condition. Therefore, it is essential to be patient.

Good nutrition is not about quick fixes; that is what crash diets are for, and they are neither sustainable nor healthy.

Nutrition cannot replace other essential aspects of well-being, such as physical activity, sleep and stress management. A perfectly balanced diet cannot build strength without exercise, nor can it reverse the negative effects of chronic sleep deprivation or unmanaged stress. All of these elements must work together to create a healthy body; food is just one part of the equation.

It is equally important to understand that nutrition cannot change your genetic makeup or reshape your natural body structure. While proper nutrition can certainly help you become a healthier version of yourself, it cannot transform you into someone else.

Additionally, no matter how nutrient-rich your meals are throughout the day, they cannot reverse the negative effects of harmful lifestyle choices such as excessive consumption of processed sugars, alcohol, smoking, or a sedentary lifestyle. Good nutrition is important, but it is most effective when combined with a balanced and healthy lifestyle.

Nutrition Comes with Energy

The sun is the primary source of energy for the Earth. Plants absorb solar energy and use it to produce the food we eat. From this food, we obtain energy, which our bodies use to function, and it is expelled in the form of sweat and breath. Thus, energy is neither created nor destroyed; it only changes form. When humans derive energy from food, it is measured in calories.

Energy is never created or destroyed, only transferred.

Energy Balance

Every nutrient or morsel of food (except plain water) contains calories. Once consumed, the body extracts energy from the food, sooner or later, depending on the type of food. The body then burns these calories as fuel to function, move and repair itself, including performing essential functions like breathing and circulation.

Calories matter!

You cannot ignore calories, regardless of whether they come from nutritious or less nutritious sources, such as coconuts or dates.

To lose, maintain or gain weight, it is essential to consume the right amount of calories.

To lose weight: Calories in < Calories out

To maintain weight: Calories in = Calories out

To gain weight: Calories in > Calories out

You do not escape calories by calling food 'natural' or 'healthy'.

When aiming to lose weight, creating a large calorie deficit is not advisable. This approach is often unsustainable and can slow your metabolism as your body adjusts to a lower-calorie intake. Therefore, when losing weight, it is important not to create a deficit greater than 10–20 per cent.

The same principle applies to weight gain. If you consume too many calories, the excess tends to result in more fat gain than muscle gain. To minimise the damage, a modest deficit or excess should be created.

Anecdote 5

Flaxseeds are healthy

About six to eight years ago, my cousin got into the flaxseed trend and learned that they are considered a superfood with numerous health benefits.

Following the lead of many well-intentioned individuals, she began consuming flaxseeds the way we typically eat *saunf* (fennel) after meals—snacking on a handful here and there, chewing on them throughout the day, and sprinkling them over her salads.

Like most people, she did not realise that these seeds are calorie-dense.

After a couple of months, she noticed that her weight was starting to creep up, even though nothing else in her routine had changed except for her constant snacking on flaxseeds. That is when she realised that just because something is healthy does not mean you can eat it in unlimited amounts.

Portion Control

The practice of eating the right amount of food to meet nutritional needs involves neither overeating nor undereating. When we start to

Overeating 'healthy' foods stalls progress just as effectively.

believe that a certain food is superior, we may end up eating more of that food, which can reduce the portion of other foods. Additionally, just because a food is considered healthy does not mean it can be eaten in unlimited quantities.

I notice that people tend to overindulge in foods like avocados, chia seeds, pumpkin seeds, nuts, dates, honey, jaggery, etc., believing they are 'healthy'.

For example, people often consume large bowls of guacamole, thinking it is 'good' for them, without realising that one medium avocado contains approximately 230–250 calories on its own.

The same goes for coconut. Just because it is 'natural', people freely eat the *malai* (cream) and pieces without recognising that one whole coconut can provide around 1,400 calories, depending on its size. Even if you divide it into 10 pieces, each piece still contains about 140 calories.

Today, cakes, cookies, and loaves of bread are being made with so-called superfoods, leading many to believe that these treats are suddenly guilt-free and healthy.

This is why awareness is important. Every food contains calories, and among all food groups, fats, nuts and seeds have the highest calorie content in the smallest volume.

When people replace sugar with alternatives like jaggery, honey or dates, they often end up overeating sweets like *mithai*s, cakes and cookies. They perceive these treats as healthy as they do not contain processed sugar.

But gram for gram, jaggery or honey provide the same number of calories as sugar.

It is important to understand that being healthy does not mean you can eat unlimited amounts of food. This distinction is crucial for maintaining your progress. Hence, portion control should be a priority. This applies not only to sugars but also to proteins and even water.

We will discuss the right portion size in detail in the subsequent chapters. For now, be cautious and avoid being misled by labels and tags that claim something is 'healthy'.

The body responds to totals first, details later.

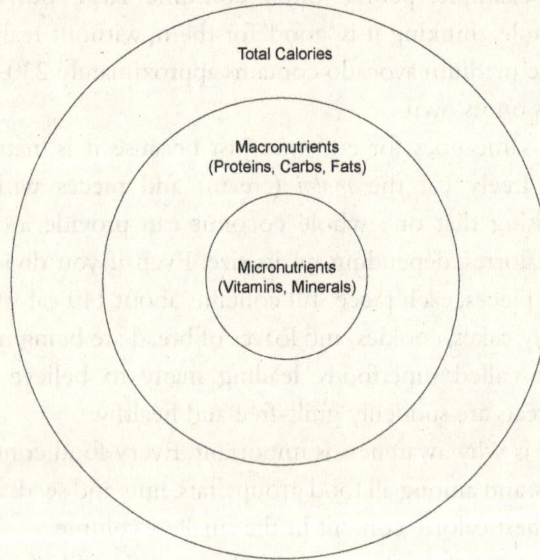

Figure 3.1: *How nutrition is often misunderstood*

Think of nutrition like this, as shown in Figure 3.1.

This is the real hierarchy:

Calories → Macros → Micros

Master the outer circles, and the inner ones will begin to fall into place.

The priority is the outermost circle: total calories. Energy balance is the foundation for every goal, whether it is fat loss, muscle gain, hormone support, or simply feeling energetic.

Regardless of how healthy a food may be, it still contains calories, and your body responds to total intake first.

Next is the macronutrient circle, which includes protein, carbohydrates, and fats. These macronutrients determine how your body utilises the calories you consume, affecting whether you maintain muscle, feel satiated, recover better, or stabilise blood sugar levels.

At number three is the smallest circle of micronutrients, which includes vitamins, minerals, phytonutrients, healthy fats like omega-3, and amino acids. These nutrients play a crucial role in supporting immunity, energy production, skin health, hair, and countless metabolic processes. While they are important, they function within the structure established by calories and macronutrients.

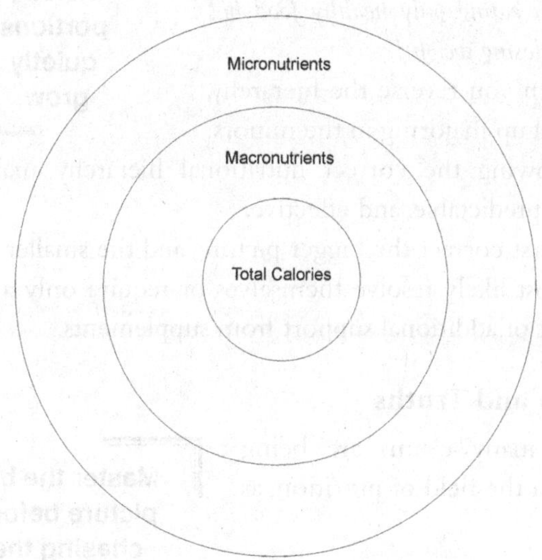

Figure 3.2: *How nutrition should be understood*

How People Commonly View Nutrition

The Reverse Hierarchy

Most people focus too much on specific details, often flipping the picture entirely. They become obsessed with the smallest components, such as micronutrients, superfoods, antioxidants, and magic pills, believing that these elements alone will transform their bodies. See Figure 3.2.

Next, they stress over macronutrients: protein, carbs, and fats. However, almost everyone ignores the foundational element: total calorie intake, which is crucial for weight change and energy balance.

This upside-down approach often leads to disappointment, confusion, and frustration, culminating in the classic statement:

When foods become 'health halos', portions quietly grow.

'I am eating only healthy food but still not losing weight!'

When you reverse the hierarchy, you end up majoring in the minors.

Following the correct nutritional hierarchy makes it simple, predictable, and effective.

So first correct the bigger picture, and the smaller issues will most likely resolve themselves or require only a small amount of additional support from supplements.

Myths and Truths

Today, many claims are being made in the field of nutrition, as

Master the big picture before chasing the fine print.

everyone tries to discover something new. Let us clarify a few points:

1. *Myth:* 'If it's healthy, it cannot become unhealthy.'
   Truth: People often believe that nutritious foods like millets, nuts, seeds, avocados, coconut, dates, and dark chocolate can be eaten freely because they are considered 'healthy'. However, anything eaten in excess can become unhealthy, especially calorie-dense foods. The healthiness of a food does not negate its calorie content.
2. *Myth:* 'A cake/cookie made with dates, whole wheat, or ragi is healthy.'
   Truth: While swapping sugar for dates or using whole wheat or ragi may add some fibre or micronutrients, it does not transform a cake into a health food. The total calories, fats and portion size often remain almost the same, and in some cases, they can even be higher due to the calorie density of dates. Essentially, a cake is still a cake. Although the ingredients might sound healthier, the overall energy content does not decrease.
3. *Myth:* 'Start your day with a litre of water.'
   Many people believe that drinking a litre of water first thing in the morning is good for digestion and detoxification.
   Truth: There is no scientific evidence to support this claim. Drinking too much water at once can overwhelm the system; what goes in quickly tends to come out quickly. Upon waking, one glass is sufficient to rehydrate. Continue to drink water steadily throughout the day.
4. *Myth:* 'Superfoods fix everything.'
   Truth: A variety of foods supports overall health. No single 'superfood' can offset a poorly structured diet

or magically cure all health issues. Regardless of the benefits of antioxidants, chia seeds, spirulina, moringa or supplements, they cannot compensate for overeating or inadequate protein consumption.

5. *Myth:* 'Chia seed water, green tea, detox water burn fat.'

   Truth: Fat loss occurs only when there is an energy balance, meaning you need to be in a calorie deficit to lose fat.

   No food or drink can directly burn fat. While some foods may assist in metabolising fat, if you do not expend that energy through physical activity, you will simply regain it. Although certain foods may improve satiety or reduce inflammation, true fat loss relies solely on maintaining an energy balance.

6. *Myth:* 'I can nullify extra calories with one intense workout.'

   Truth: Many people believe that a strong workout can cancel out the effects of overeating. This is not true. Your body does not operate like a calculator; you can exhaust yourself long before you manage to burn off the calories from a binge. One workout cannot make up for repeated high-calorie intake. While physical activity is beneficial for health, it cannot override your body's overall energy balance.

7. *Myth:* 'You do not need to think about calories if you are active.'

   Truth: While movement is beneficial, being active does not negate the effects of overeating.

   Even athletes can gain fat if they disregard their energy intake.

Food works best as support, not as a solution to everything.

To Reiterate

- There are no superfoods.
- All foods come with energy.
- Calories matter. Energy balance matters.
- Portion control should be the priority.
- Everything real is healthy. Portion makes the poison.

A Note from Me to You

In a world obsessed with 'superfoods', fancy diets and quick fixes, I want you to remember something simple: your body runs on balance, not hype. No single food will transform your health, and no single meal will derail it. What truly creates change is an energy balance: how much you take in versus how much you use, and the portions you consistently choose. My intention with this book is to help you build a relationship with food that feels supportive, sustainable, and grounded in real science rather than trends.

Habit 3

From finding 'good' in others to becoming non-judgemental towards your food

Wake up to eat.

Eat to nourish your body.

Eat to celebrate life.

Eat with gratitude, not judgement.

Stop labelling your food as 'good' or 'bad', 'junk', 'cheat' or even 'healthy'. Everything real and edible is already good. Most importantly, do not fear any food.

Record your daily meals in the food log without guilt or pride. Just note what you eat, exactly as it is, with no deliberate changes, no hiding, and no overthinking. Simply observe and record, as explained in the previous chapter.

Get the foundation right, and the details become manageable.

4

Hydration: The Zero-Calorie Drink

WATER IS THE ONLY drink we truly need: plain, simple water. Every other beverage we consume is influenced by culture, climate, taste or habit. The beauty of water lies in its simplicity.

> **Water is not just a drink. It is the medium in which life runs.**

Water is a zero-calorie drink!

Water is often overlooked as a 'nutrient', but it is the most important one because every chemical reaction in the body requires it. Without it, nothing functions efficiently. The human body consists of 55 per cent to 80 per cent water, depending on factors such as age, gender and body composition.

How Much Water Do We Need?

Fluid needs vary with body size, activity level, climate, diet, and age; therefore, there is no universal recommendation like 'eight glasses a day'. A simple and practical method to assess hydration for most people is to check the colour of their urine.

> **Hydration is personal, not prescriptive.**

- Dark yellow: likely dehydration
- Pale yellow: generally adequate hydration
- Clear/white: often associated with over-hydration

However, it is important to interpret urine colour in context. The first urine of the morning tends to be darker because you have not consumed fluids for several hours. This natural concentration reflects the body's overnight water conservation process and is not a sign of dehydration. Additionally, factors such as a higher intake of salty or high-protein meals, intense exercise and certain supplements or medications can temporarily concentrate urine. This is a normal physiological response and does not automatically indicate inadequate hydration.

What matters most is the colour of your urine after your first few glasses of water and throughout the day. This should be considered alongside your lifestyle, environment, activity level, and actual fluid intake.

Urine colour is a useful guide, but like all body signals, it must be evaluated in context rather than used in isolation.

A word of caution: urine colour is a guide, not an absolute rule.

While urine colour is a reliable real-time indicator of hydration for most people, it is still not absolute for everyone. Some individuals may have pale or even clear urine despite not drinking much water. This is especially true for those whose circadian rhythms are disrupted, such as night-shift workers. Additionally, people taking electrolytes without enough water may also experience pale-coloured urine, as high sodium or potassium levels can temporarily draw water into the urine.

Diet also plays a significant role in urine concentration. Factors such as low salt or low protein intake, high water content in foods, and frequent caffeine consumption can all lead to more diluted urine. Additionally, natural variations in kidney efficiency introduce further differences in urine concentration.

Urine colour is a helpful indicator of hydration and should not be interpreted in isolation. To get an accurate understanding of your hydration needs, consider your overall fluid intake, lifestyle, activity level, and environment.

Urine colour is a signal, not a verdict.

Anecdote 6

When clear urine misleads

One of my clients is a thirty-two-year-old doctor who works in a busy government hospital. She often believed she was well-hydrated, despite only drinking about 1 litre of water a day. Interestingly, her urine was consistently pale or almost clear.

Context matters more than appearances.

Due to emergency calls, unpredictable schedules, and at least one 24-hour duty every week, she rarely had the opportunity to drink enough water. This may have begun with her avoiding water due to limited access to clean toilets, which gradually became a habit. Because her urine appeared clear, she assumed she was 'doing fine'.

Upon further investigation, we found that her night duties and irregular sleep patterns were disrupting her natural circadian rhythm. This disruption can affect the body's ability to regulate urine concentration. As a result, her urine appeared clear despite a low overall fluid intake. Add to this long gaps between meals, a low-salt diet, and the regular consumption of caffeine to stay awake, which contributed to the situation. It became clear that urine colour alone was an unreliable indicator of her hydration status.

She was not adequately hydrated; her body just was not showing this in the usual way.

This experience serves as a reminder that for some individuals, especially shift workers, clear urine can be misleading and that hydration should be assessed more holistically.

Why Does Hydration Matter So Much?

When you are well hydrated, your body runs like a lubricated machine.

Hydration does not just prevent thirst; it protects function.

- **Energy and metabolism:** Water plays a crucial role in helping cells produce energy efficiently. It supports metabolic rates and ensures oxygen and nutrients are circulated smoothly throughout the body, reducing strain on the heart.
- **Headache and migraine:** Mild dehydration or long intervals without fluid intake can cause the tissues surrounding the brain to temporarily shrink. This shrinkage can activate pain receptors, potentially leading to headaches or triggering migraines in individuals who are prone to them.
- **Fatigue prevention:** Dehydration makes your heart work harder, which consumes more energy and can leave you feeling drained.
- **Digestion and detox:** Water plays a vital role in supporting healthy digestion, maintaining regular bowel movements, and helping to flush out waste products. This means that staying hydrated is essential for a healthy gut and urinary system.
- **Craving control:** Often, what we perceive as a snack craving is actually just mild dehydration. Drinking

water regularly can help reduce unnecessary cravings for sugar and salt.

- **Mood and focus:** Mild dehydration, resulting in a 1–2 per cent loss of body weight, can impair memory, concentration and mood stability.

Tip: For those watching their weight, water is a silent ally. Drinking it before and during meals, as well as throughout the day, reduces cravings and helps maintain control over portion sizes.

Hydration and Physical Performance

Your muscles consist of nearly 70–75 per cent water. Proper hydration enables muscles to contract and relax efficiently during physical activity. Even a small decrease in hydration can reduce endurance, strength and power output.

Dehydration not only leads to fatigue but also increases the risk of several other issues, including the following:

- Muscle cramps
- Joint stiffness
- Impaired heat regulation (increasing the risk of heat stroke)
- Increased strain on the cardiovascular system

Tip: For athletes or anyone exercising in hot climates, such as hot yoga or steam and sauna rooms, staying hydrated is not optional; it enhances performance and serves as a crucial safety net.

The Role of Electrolytes

While water is foundational, proper hydration is more than just H_2O. Your body also needs electrolytes, such as sodium, potassium, magnesium and chloride. These minerals help maintain fluid balance between cells, regulate nerve function, and control muscle contractions.

- Sodium helps regulate blood pressure and maintain fluid balance.
- Potassium counteracts sodium, relaxes blood vessels and promotes heart health.
- Magnesium is essential for muscle relaxation and helps prevent cramps.
- Chloride assists in balancing acids and bases in the body.

Sweating, illness, or intense exercise can deplete electrolytes, which is why replenishing them is just as important as staying hydrated. In most cases, regular home-cooked meals provide sufficient electrolytes. Foods such as coconut water, buttermilk, fruits and vegetables can also help restore electrolyte balance naturally, eliminating the need for commercial sports drinks. For typical exercise sessions lasting up to an hour, you generally do not need additional electrolytes or sports drinks.

Hydration is balance, not just volume.

However, this does not mean supplemental electrolytes are always unnecessary. In certain cases, they become important. For example, a marathon runner may find it difficult to eat solid food during the race, as swallowing and digestion can be challenging during prolonged, intense activity. In such situations, electrolyte supplements help maintain fluid balance, prevent cramps, and support overall performance. Similarly, during diarrhoea, the body loses significant amounts of electrolytes through frequent, watery stools, making electrolyte-rich oral rehydration solutions necessary for proper recovery.

Signs of Dehydration

The colour of the urine is the simplest indicator of dehydration, but there are other signs to watch for, including:

- Dry mouth and lips
- Headaches or dizziness
- Constipation
- Dark circles under the eyes or tired eyes
- Poor skin elasticity
- Low energy and irritability

Chronic dehydration is quiet but costly.

Chronic, low-grade dehydration is surprisingly common, especially among older adults, who may not feel thirst as strongly.

Special Hydration Needs

- **Children:** Active kids can lose fluids quickly due to play and sweating. Encourage them to take frequent sips of water rather than waiting until they feel thirsty.
- **Older adults:** The sensation of thirst often declines with age. It is important for them to drink consciously, even when they do not feel thirsty.
- **Athletes and active individuals:** They require both water and electrolytes. It is crucial to hydrate before and during physical activity.
- **Hot and humid climates:** In such conditions, sweat loss increases, making it important to consume water and electrolyte-rich foods.

- **Illness:** Conditions like fever, diarrhoea or vomiting can lead to severe fluid loss. Rehydration solutions or broths can help restore fluid balance.

Hydrating Beyond Water

While plain water should be your primary choice for hydration, other fluids can also contribute significantly:

- Herbal teas
- Coconut water
- Buttermilk (*chaas*)
- Soups and broths
- Fruits and vegetables (like watermelon, cucumber and oranges)

Caffeinated beverages like tea and coffee also count towards hydration. While caffeine has a mild diuretic effect, the water content in these drinks typically outweighs the negative effect, unless consumed in excessive amounts.

Water and Weight Management

For those aiming for weight loss or maintenance, hydration is an often-overlooked tool. Drinking water:

- helps prevent confusing thirst with hunger;
- keeps cravings at bay;
- improves workout efficiency, allowing you to burn more calories; and
- supports fat metabolism, as lipolysis requires water.

Even mild dehydration can slow metabolism, so maintaining proper hydration boosts the body's efficiency in burning fat.

More is not always better, even with water.

Over-hydration: yes, it is possible

While rare, it is indeed possible to drink too much water, which can lead to hyponatremia, a condition characterised by dangerously low sodium levels. This is often observed in endurance athletes who consume excessive amounts of water without replenishing their electrolytes. Symptoms of over-hydration include nausea, confusion, muscle weakness and, in extreme cases, seizures.

Hyponatremia is not caused by drinking a little extra water; rather, it is a rare condition that occurs when a person consumes excessive amounts of water—usually over 4–5 litres in just a couple of hours—without adequate sodium replacement. This condition arises when serum sodium levels fall below 135 mmol/litre due to excessive water intake. Your kidneys can excrete roughly 0.8–1.0 litres of water per hour. In short, your body is well-equipped to maintain balance, so do not be afraid of water; a little extra water here and there does not harm.

Tip: When sweating heavily for extended periods (especially over an hour), balance water intake with electrolyte replacement.

Hydration works best as a habit, not a rule.

A note of caution: while coconut water is often perceived as universally healthy, it should still be consumed mindfully. It is relatively high in potassium and low in sodium. Excessive intake—particularly in individuals with low blood pressure, high sweat losses, kidney issues or low overall sodium intake—can lead to an electrolyte imbalance, dizziness or headaches. As with all foods, moderation is the key, not hype.

A Practical Hydration Guide

From a coaching perspective, a daily intake of about 2 litres is considered the minimum baseline for most adults. However, those who are active, who consume higher amounts of protein or fibre, or who have greater physiological demands, often benefit from a fluid intake of 2.5–3.5 litres. This guideline is not prescriptive but rather practical, allowing for daily adjustments based on factors such as urine colour, thirst, energy levels and overall performance.

Building Your Hydration Mindset

Hydration should not just be a task to complete; it should be a daily habit to nurture. Think of water as the 'oil' for your body's machinery. Just as a machine runs smoothly when it is regularly oiled, your body functions best when it is consistently hydrated.

If you struggle to drink enough water, build gradually. Set reminders, take small sips, and slowly increase your intake. Over time, staying hydrated will become a natural habit.

Final Thoughts

Water is the simplest, cheapest, and most powerful wellness tool we have, yet it is often ignored. Staying hydrated helps maintain stable energy levels, supports heart health, sharpens mental clarity, reduces cravings, keeps skin supple and improves workout performance.

Ignore the myths and pay attention to your body. Remember: it is not about overwhelming yourself with litres of water but about maintaining steady, mindful hydration throughout the day.

Start with that one glass of water in the morning; sip it mindfully and let water nourish every cell in your body.

Drink steadily. Stay aware. Let water do its work quietly.

Myths and Truths

The world of health is filled with various beliefs and myths that stem from old theories and cultural practices. If that was not enough, today everyone seems to be vying to share unique perspectives that catch people's attention. Hydration is no exception. So let us clear a few.

1. *Myth:* 'Do not drink water with meals.'
   This is perhaps the most common myth. Some people claim it dilutes gastric juices and interferes with digestion.
   Truth: No evidence supports this claim. In fact, water helps soften food and aids digestion. A 2021 study found that drinking water before meals was linked to lower body weight, reduced waist circumference, and improved blood sugar and lipid levels in people with Type 2 diabetes.[1]
   So, feel free to drink water before, during or after meals—whenever you like it.
2. *Myth:* 'You must drink 3 to 4 litres of water every day, no exceptions.'
   Truth: Hydration needs vary from person to person. A petite woman working in an air-conditioned office will require less water than a tall athlete training outdoors in humid conditions.

   Pay attention to your body, check your urine colour, and adjust your water intake accordingly.

3. *Myth:* 'Start your day with a litre of water.'
   Some people believe that drinking a large amount of water in the morning is good for digestion and detoxification.
   Truth: There is no scientific evidence to support this claim. Drinking too much water at once can overwhelm your system. What you take in quickly will also exit quickly.
   Upon waking, one glass of water is sufficient to rehydrate. After that, it is best to continue drinking steadily throughout the day.
4. *Myth:* 'Drinking water during exercise will make you sick.'
   A common belief, especially in India, is that if you are sweating and feeling hot from exercising, drinking water, especially cold water, can create a clash of temperatures ('*thande–garam ka paleta*') that can make you ill.
   Truth: There is no scientific evidence to support this claim. On the contrary, not drinking water while exercising increases the risk of dehydration, cramps, dizziness, and even heat stroke. Your body is well-equipped to handle cold water, even when you are warm; in fact, it actually helps regulate your temperature and prevents overheating. The key is moderation: sip small amounts of room-temperature or cold water during your workouts, and your body will thank you.
5. *Myth:* 'Only plain water counts.'
   Truth: Hydration can also come from food and other fluids. Soups, fruits, vegetables, milk, yoghurt, tea, coffee and *dal*s all contribute to hydration.

6. *Myth:* 'You should always drink only warm water; cold water is harmful.'

   Ayurveda often recommends drinking warm water to improve digestion and to maintain balance.

   Truth: Modern nutrition does not restrict water temperature. In reality, there is no scientific evidence that cold or room-temperature water is harmful. Even icy cold water does not directly harm the throat; its effects are more related to your overall immunity and individual comfort. Ultimately, the best water temperature is simply the one that feels most comfortable to you.
7. *Myth:* 'You need "body-like pH" water to stay healthy.'

   Many premium waters claim to match the body's pH or promise special benefits because they are more alkaline.

   Truth: Your body already regulates its own pH with incredible precision, regardless of the type of water you drink. The pH of water is neutralised by stomach acid, and the kidneys and lungs manage the rest. There is no strong scientific evidence that alkaline, black or 'Spring/Himalayan' water offers any superior health benefits compared to clean, regular water. While hydration is crucial, the pH level of your water is not. However, people with acid reflux may experience temporary relief when drinking slightly alkaline water.

To Reiterate

- There is no universal 'eight glasses a day' rule: hydration needs vary widely.
- Urine colour serves as a practical, real-time indicator of hydration, but it should be interpreted within the right context.
- Shift workers, especially those with irregular sleep cycles, may not exhibit the typical urine colour cues related to hydration.

- Dehydration frequently triggers headaches and migraines, and can easily go unnoticed.
- Consistent, mindful fluid intake can prevent cravings.

A Note from Me to You

Anything new tends to catch people's fancy, whether it is alkaline water, black water, energy drinks or electrolyte tablets. However, your body operates best on balance, not on novelty. Most people function perfectly well with regular, consistent hydration and do not need special waters or added electrolytes—save those for individuals who genuinely require them.

If you frequently experience headaches or cravings, start by examining your hydration habits. Sometimes, simply drinking water steadily throughout the day can make a meaningful difference. This small habit often provides surprisingly big relief.

As a practical guideline, I generally recommend aiming for a little over 2.5 litres of water a day, depending on your body size, activity level, climate, and lifestyle. This is a starting point, not a strict rule. Listen to your body and adjust your intake as needed.

Habit 4

Sip more water throughout the day

Practical hydration habits

If you struggle to drink enough water, here are some helpful tips:

- Carry a bottle with you: a visible cue helps.
- Set hourly reminders: especially if you tend to forget to hydrate.
- Start small: even sipping a little water adds up. Gradually work your way up to half a glass and then a full cup.

- Flavour naturally: if you find plain water unappealing, try adding lemon, cucumber, or mint. However, it is beneficial to eventually develop a habit of drinking plain water.
- Hydrate smartly: start your day with a glass of water and drink at regular intervals throughout the day. Reduce your intake closer to bedtime to avoid waking up at night to use the washroom.

Remember, hydration is less about 'gulping a lot at once' and more about steady sipping throughout the day.

5

Breakfast: The First Meal of the Day Matters

WHEN YOU ARE UNSURE what to do, look to nature for guidance. A simple rule to follow is to align your eating patterns with the sun.

Start by synchronising your body clock with the natural day. As the sun rises, it is time for you to wake up and be active, rather than slipping back into sleep. To function effectively throughout the day, you need fuel. Remember that energy is not created; it is exchanged, and food is your primary source of energy.

For many people, especially those who train early or experience chronic stress, eating within 30–45 minutes of waking up can be beneficial.[1] As the sun reaches its highest point in the sky, it is time for your main meal. Then, as daylight begins to fade, have your last substantial meal of the day. Your final meal, or supper, can be a light snack.

Your body is like a day-shift worker. It is designed to wake, eat, move, and digest best when there is daylight.

If I could recommend a habit to everyone, it would be this: eat something within 30–45 minutes of waking up.

Let us dig deeper into how your body actually prefers to align itself with the sun, meaning the circadian rhythm.

Breakfast and the Body's 'Power-Save Mode'

One of the most fascinating things about the human body is how it manages energy during sleep and wakefulness. Each night, when we go to bed, we enter a natural fasting period. For six to eight hours, sometimes longer, the body goes without food.

Yet, amazingly, it still keeps us alive and functioning, maintaining our heartbeat, breathing, repair processes, and even growth.

When morning arrives, a key hormone is released to awaken us: cortisol, the most feared hormone.

Cortisol

Cortisol is often viewed as the enemy, yet it is one of the most vital and essential hormones in our bodies.

Before discussing its awakening response, I want you to understand that this hormone can work to your advantage if you learn to balance it through your behaviour.

Cortisol is not a villain; it is your internal alarm clock and fuel manager.

You cannot directly control your hormones, but you can support your body's ability to manage and balance them efficiently through your behaviour, thoughts, habits, and activities.

It is this very hormone that causes you to move or react in emergencies. When cortisol activates during danger, it can make you run faster than you ever imagined.

So, do not fear cortisol; understand it. Equip yourself with the knowledge to let it work at its natural pace.

Your body starts waking you up before you open your eyes.

Cortisol Awakening

While you are asleep, your circadian rhythm is already preparing your body for the day ahead. Later in the night, cortisol gradually rises, starting slowly at first and then more significantly as morning approaches.

This early-morning rise helps the body shift from rest to alertness: it signals metabolism, primes the liver to release glucose for morning energy, and supports alertness. This is the cortisol awakening response (CAR)[2], helping you move from recovery mode to action mode.

So, it is not the alarm clock that wakes your physiology; your body is already waking up before it goes off.

Now, here is where food, especially breakfast timing, comes into play. If fasting continues, meaning you do not eat, the body keeps making the liver release glucose through gluconeogenesis, providing energy to keep you going. While this keeps you functional, it also keeps the body in a stress-driven, conservation mode rather than allowing

If food does not come in, the body makes its own fuel to keep you moving.

it to switch into a fed, fuel-available state. There is a simple way to see this.

The 'Power-Saving Mode' Metaphor

I will emphasise that this is a metaphor I created to simplify. It is not a literal medical fact.

When you do not eat anything during the first hour of waking, you indirectly signal to your body that there is a shortage of food: 'Please manage on your own.'

In other words, the body sees it as a signal: 'There is not enough fuel right now.'

So, just like your smartphone, it activates its power-saving mode.

What Happens in Power-Saving Mode?

When your phone enters power-saving mode, the open app continues to work, but other background activities are temporarily paused, right?

Your body functions the same way. It is incredibly loyal to you, with its first priority being to keep you alive.

The body prioritises energy for essential functions, especially the brain, over performance and repair. To accomplish this, muscles temporarily become less responsive and less efficient at absorbing sugar, which can make you feel less energetic and discourage unnecessary movement. However, since it is morning and most of us are in a hurry, the body still releases glucose from the liver, providing just enough for survival, not optimal functioning.

It also begins to limit energy and nutrients to areas that are not essential for immediate survival, such as hair, skin, and nails. Over time, chronic under-fuelling can increase protein breakdown and result in dull skin, slower nail growth, or hair issues.

Now, does skipping breakfast once in a while cause hair loss? Of course not. That is not how physiology works in the short term. But this metaphor is meant to explain that the body is constantly assessing: 'Do we have enough fuel to support not just survival, but thriving?'

> **Your body always feeds survival first; everything else gets what is left.**

What Keeps You Alive?

Your internal systems: the vital organs.

These are the parts of your body that operate automatically, without conscious control: your brain, heart, lungs, liver, kidneys and gut. Keeping these systems functioning is the body's top priority, even when energy is limited.

So, the body provides just enough energy to keep these organs functioning at a basic level, though they may not operate optimally when the body is under-fuelled.

> **Early food tells the body: 'You do not have to struggle today.'**

What Should You Do?

Give your body a quick boost of calories. Remember, calories are energy: fuel for the body.

A simple fruit can be a gentle way to break the fast. Carbohydrates from fruit quickly raise blood glucose, triggering insulin release. Do not confuse this with a sugar spike; this rise is a natural physiological response to food and should not be feared.

While cortisol and insulin are not exact opposites, they work together in balance. Cortisol raises blood glucose by signalling the liver to release it, which is helpful in short bursts but causes stress if it lasts too long. Insulin, on the other hand, helps glucose from food enter the cells, where it can be used for energy, movement and repair.

Eating early signals the body that external fuel is available. This reduces reliance on cortisol-driven glucose release and allows insulin to work more effectively, helping the body transition from survival mode to a fed, fuel-available state.

Some people think that 'using stored glucose' will automatically help burn fat, but the body is much smarter than we often realise.As fasting continues, the body patiently waits for the right moment to restore energy balance, often by increasing hunger, fatigue and cravings for sweet or salty foods later in the day.

Many intermittent fasting enthusiasts might disagree with this view. However, it is important to remember that the body's primary goal is survival, not optimisation. Extended fasting periods can make it harder to keep a positive nitrogen balance, especially if overall protein intake is insufficient.

When the body waits too long for fuel, it asks louder later.

Cortisol and Insulin: Partners, Not Enemies

Let us clarify this once more: cortisol is not a 'bad' hormone. It is often labelled the stress hormone, but that description is incomplete. Without cortisol, you would not wake up, mobilise energy or respond to challenges.

Insulin is not the enemy either; it is the hormone that helps your cells to use glucose for energy. Problems arise only when either cortisol or insulin remains chronically elevated over time, even when the body no longer needs that response.

So, when I say fruit helps control cortisol, I do not mean that eating fruit magically lowers stress. I mean that feeding the body after an overnight fast, particularly with carbohydrates first, then some protein, sends a clear message to the system: 'Fuel is available. No need to stay on high alert.'

Sometimes the body does not need more discipline; it needs safety.

Respect Your Body's Signals

The question is not really whether breakfast is good or bad. It is whether delaying food aligns with your biology or works against it. There is no one-size-fits-all rule. Some people feel fine delaying their first meal, while others function better with early nourishment.

However, based on my experience, eating something within the first hour of waking up often helps people feel more stable, less reactive and more energised as the day progresses, especially women and those coping with fatigue, hormonal shifts or thyroid imbalances.[3]

Bodies under stress respond better to reassurance than restriction.

Meal timing, including breakfast, affects circadian signalling that helps regulate the sleep–wake cycle.[4]

Practical Takeaways

So, what should you do with all this information?

- If you feel sluggish, anxious, or overly hungry later in the day, try eating breakfast within 30 to 60 minutes of waking up. Even something as small as half a banana, followed by yoghurt or milk, can help.
- If you are comfortable delaying food and your energy, hormones, and digestion are stable, that is fine too. There is no universal rule. However, I recommend trying the above approach for a month to see how your body reacts.
- Balance matters. A good breakfast should include some carbohydrates (fruit, whole grains), protein (eggs, yoghurt, or protein powder) and healthy fats (seeds, nuts, avocado or the fat used in cooking).

Anecdote 7

When her body finally felt safe

One of my clients, a forty-six-year-old athlete and an avid tennis player, came to me feeling completely frustrated. She had worked with multiple dietitians and nutritionists over the years, yet nothing seemed to change: her hypothyroid symptoms persisted, her recovery was slow, and her weight refused to shift.

When I reviewed her routine, the problem became clear.

She woke up every morning at 4:00 or 4:30 a.m., laced her shoes, and went straight to the tennis court. She played intensely for an hour to an hour and a half before eating anything. Then she came home, finally ate breakfast and went about her day, all while maintaining a strict calorie deficit that had been prescribed to her for months, with a few no-salt days and weeks without grains.

When I sat her down and gently explained what was happening, I told her, 'Your body has been running in survival mode.' She was devastated to hear this.

She was already battling a slow metabolism caused by hypothyroidism. However, she was also pushing her body into an emergency state every morning by engaging in high-intensity sports without any fuel intake. The severe calorie deficit only worsened her recovery, leading to extreme soreness, overstressed systems, and undernourishment.

Over the next six weeks, I had to reverse diet her. The first thing I introduced was a fruit and a protein supplement in the morning. Within a week, she told me her soreness had gone away. She was playing better and even giving the men in the game a good fight.

I gradually increased her food intake, reassuring her that nothing 'bad' would happen, teaching her that her body needed to feel safe again. She trusted me, and I told her, 'I just want you to relax and eat. I am here. You are not alone in this process.'

Twenty days into this plan, she left for a holiday. I told her to eat whatever she felt like eating, no restrictions. She was confused, but did so. She ate freely (though being an athlete, she ate nourishing food most of the time), moved joyfully, slept deeply, and simply allowed herself to be happy.

When she returned, her waist was 1–1.5 inches smaller, even though we had increased her calorie intake rather than cutting it.

What changed? Safety.

Her body finally relaxed from its survival mode. Her stress response calmed down. Her system shifted out of chronic stress. Her metabolism responded. Her body realised: Yes, I can breathe now. I am safe.

And that is when her progress began. Yes, slow by her standards, but still moving in the right direction.

Coaching Perspective

In my practice, I have learned that simple metaphors, such as the body going into a power-saving mode, help people without a scientific background understand what is happening inside them. It is not a literal shutdown but a practical way to explain how eating early in the day can set the tone for more stable energy, mood and long-term health.

My role as a coach is to turn both science and lived observations into simple guidance you can follow. You can try it out, watch how your body reacts, and make adjustments as needed.

Because ultimately, the best diet is not the one found in textbooks; it is the one that works for your body.

Myths and Truths

1. *Myth:* 'Cortisol is a bad hormone and must be lowered.'
   Truth: Cortisol is essential for waking up, mobilising energy and keeping you alive. Problems arise only when it stays chronically elevated for a long time. Morning cortisol is a healthy physiological response.
2. *Myth:* 'Skipping breakfast boosts metabolism because it burns stored fat.'
   Truth: Extended morning fasting increases reliance on liver-driven glucose release. While this aids survival, it may lower energy, boost cravings later, and is not ideal for many people, especially women.
3. *Myth:* 'Insulin spikes in the morning are harmful.'
   Truth: A slight increase in insulin after breakfast is normal and beneficial. It signals the body that fuel is available, supports hormonal balance, reduces unnecessary cortisol-driven glucose release, and allows the body to transition from a stress-driven, fasted state to a fed, fuel-available state.
4. *Myth:* 'Breakfast is either essential for everyone or unnecessary for everyone.'
   Truth: There is no one-size-fits-all solution. But if your energy, mood, cravings, or hormones feel off, trying to

eat within 30–45 minutes of waking up can be a powerful experiment.

5. *Myth:* 'The body will function at its best even if you skip early food, as long as calories are balanced.'
   Truth: Your body prioritises survival first. Without early fuel, it conserves energy for essential organs, not optimisation, which may show up as reduced energy, lower productivity or skin/hair changes over time.
6. *Myth:* 'Eating a fruit early in the morning is dangerous.'
   Truth: For most people, fruit is one of the gentlest ways to break an overnight fast; it fits well with your circadian rhythm and supports natural glucose regulation.

The only situations where timing might need adjustment are uncontrolled diabetes, severe reactive hypoglycaemia, or when advised by a clinician for specific medical reasons. Even then, fruit is not 'dangerous'; it just needs pairing with protein or fat.

To Reiterate

- Your body prioritises survival, not optimisation.
- Your body wakes up before you do, guided by CAR.
- Eating within 30–45 minutes of waking provides external fuel when your system needs it most.
- Early food reduces reliance on liver-driven glucose and supports smoother hormonal balance.
- Breakfast timing influences circadian rhythm, metabolism, and even melatonin regulation.
- A small first meal is enough: fruit, yoghurt, milk, or a light carb and protein combination.
- Women and those with fatigue or thyroid issues often respond best to early nourishment.

- Skipping early food can keep the body in 'energy conservation mode', affecting vitality.
- The body listens to actions and cues, not commands.
- The body responds through energy, efficiency, sleep, recovery, hormones and symptoms; we just need to learn to listen to it.
- There is no universal rule: try to see how your body responds.
- The best diet is not the most popular one; it is the one that matches your biology.

A Note from Me to You

For years, I have watched people struggle with energy crashes, cravings, mood swings, and hormonal symptoms, often without realising that something as simple as when they eat their first meal can make a big difference.

This chapter is not about telling you what is 'right' or 'wrong'.

It is about helping you understand your body's natural rhythm, the one it has been following since long before diets and trends existed.

I want you to understand how nature and science are intertwined. We just need to 'listen' to our own signals and then apply science to them, experimenting gently. You do not need perfection; you just need alignment.

Whether you choose to eat early or explore fasting, let it be a decision made with awareness, not pressure.

Your body speaks.

You just need to listen.

Understanding the body does not require medical jargon, just the right lens.

Habit 5

Eat within the first 30–45 minutes of waking up

It is best to start your day with a fruit—any fruit you like. Pick one that makes you happy. It could be a mango, a banana, or whatever feels easiest for you. If cutting or chopping feels like a hassle, opt for something simple like a banana, grapes, strawberries, blueberries, a small apple or an orange. Choose what is most convenient and comfortable for you.

One thing to remember: when you change your morning habits, especially if you are not used to eating early, your body might initially push back. You might feel mild discomfort, like gas or heartburn, a couple of hours after eating. This is because the body does not like sudden changes.

Do not worry; this is normal. The key is persistence and trying new things. If a fruit causes discomfort, try a different fruit the next day. Keep this up for a few days. By the third or fourth day, your body usually begins to adjust and accept the fruit that works best for you.

Once you find a fruit that suits you, stick with it for a few days. Then, you can even try the fruit that caused issues on day one again. There is a good chance your body will now accept it. If it still causes discomfort, repeat the process with gradual adjustments.

Over time, as your body recognises your consistency and persistence, it will adapt. This way, your morning fruit habit becomes smooth, easy and enjoyable.

6

Balanced Meal Frequency

Eat Four to Six Meals a Day

Again, this is not set in stone. Some people eat one meal a day, others eat two, and others have more.

When I say 'four to six meals a day', I do not mean six large plates of food.

What counts as a meal?

Many people think of a meal as a big plate of food, often overlooking their cups of tea or coffee. But from a physiological standpoint, even a small caloric intake qualifies as a meal.[1]

> **Even small amounts of food signal the body to start digestion and energy management.**

The Science Behind a Meal

When calories, even in small amounts, enter your system, your body initiates a chemical response:

- Insulin levels rise to help manage the incoming glucose.
- Digestive enzymes and stomach acid increase to break down the food.
- The metabolic cycle shifts into what is known as 'fed mode'.

Even the smallest calorie triggers a response.

Even something that seems harmless, like a splash of milk in your coffee, a spoon of nut butter, or a few almonds, breaks your fast or counts as a mini-meal.

Being aware of this helps you plan better. Instead of mindlessly snacking, organise your meals so that each eating occasion has a purpose. Ask yourself: Am I feeding hunger, habit or emotion right now?

'Four to six meals a day' simply means spreading your daily nutrition across the day in a way that fits your lifestyle and keeps your metabolism active.

Meal Structure

For most people, a realistic structure appears as follows:

- Meal 1: Pre-workout nutrition, in case training is early in the morning (or breakfast, as applicable)
- Meal 2: Breakfast (or mid-morning snack, as applicable)
- Meal 3: Mid-morning snack (or lunch, if applicable)
- Meal 4: Lunch (or an early evening snack, if there is a long gap)
- Meal 5: Evening meal (or dinner, as required)
- Meal 6: Supper or snack (optional, if required)

Six is the upper limit.[2] Most people do well with four to five structured eating occasions, and the sixth usually only fits if there is an early-morning or late-evening workout.

But let us say you are someone who cannot eat too many meals. In that case, I would recommend having at least three meals. You can combine snacks with your main meals and still get all the nutrition you need. Instead of spreading your daily calories over four to five meals, you are dividing them into three meals.

The key is consistency. Eating almost at the same time each day helps regulate your circadian rhythm, improves digestion, and can help your body better manage cortisol and insulin. The body thrives on discipline. When you eat irregularly, skipping meals one day and overeating the next, your metabolism, hormones, and digestion struggle to stay balanced.

Eat by the Clock, Not Just by Hunger

We often hear, 'Eat only when you are hungry.'

Our body runs on an internal clock, and eating at regular times helps keep this clock in sync.

But here is the catch: this works perfectly only if your hunger cues are reliable. For many people, especially those working long hours, having erratic schedules, or dealing with chronic stress, hunger cues can become completely out of sync with their body's actual energy needs.

That is where the idea of eating by the clock comes in. When you eat at roughly the same times every day, your body begins to anticipate those timings. Over time, hunger cues begin to appear on a schedule, and that becomes a routine. It is like training your metabolism to stay balanced, not fluctuating between starvation and overeating.

If you wait to eat until you are really starving, several things could happen:

- You might end up overeating because your body tries to compensate for lost energy, and you eat out of pity for not having eaten in a long time, which leads to eating more. You see this as a reward for going hungry for so long.

- You tend to grab whatever is most convenient, often sugar or refined carbs. If that food takes longer to prepare or even heat, you might get so hungry that you eat ready-to-eat food to pass the immediate hunger.

Long gaps without food can make the body feel stressed, increasing stress hormone levels.

- Your stress hormones, like cortisol, increase because the body perceives food scarcity as a threat. And if this becomes a pattern, your body keeps your cortisol levels high over time.

The Three- to Four-Hour Rule

Now, let us discuss the intervals between meals.

Eating every three to four hours helps keep your blood sugar stable, your mood even, and your energy consistent throughout the day. Think of it as fuelling your body with required, regular doses instead of waiting for your tank to run empty and refilling it all at once.

I recommend keeping it between three and four hours. Try to maintain at least a two-hour gap. Avoid grazing throughout the day or going long periods without eating. So, avoid eating within two hours of a meal, and try not to extend it much beyond four hours. For most people, a three- to four-hour gap works well.

Here is why.

Eating at regular intervals helps prevent sharp drops and spikes in energy.

If you eat again too soon, say within an hour or two of your last bite, your digestive system never gets a break. Constant grazing keeps insulin levels elevated, which can slow down fat metabolism and cause fatigue or bloating. On the other hand, if you extend the gap beyond four hours, your blood sugar can drop too low, leading to irritability, cravings, and poor food choices later.[3]

A three- to four-hour window strikes the perfect balance, giving your gut time to digest and absorb nutrients while ensuring your brain and muscles receive a steady supply of energy.

So, if you finish breakfast between 7:00 and 8:00 a.m., your mid-morning snack should ideally be around 11:00 or 12 noon, with lunch by 2:00 or 4:00 p.m., and so on. This pattern helps regulate hunger and fullness signals and prevents you from reaching the point where you could 'eat anything in sight'.

If you, let us say, enjoy a cup of tea or coffee after a meal, you can wait about 30 minutes before having that beverage and consider it part of the meal beforehand. Your eating time should start from the end of this tea or coffee. Try to avoid drinking any beverages other than water before a meal, as it can suppress your appetite, and we want you to eat.

So, no snacking in between. If you are drinking a calorie-containing drink, munching on a handful of nuts, chips, or sneaking in a small piece of chocolate, that is technically another meal.

Ideally, every meal must have protein.

Now, this is a principle I strongly emphasise: every meal must include a protein source or be a complete meal. If that is not possible, at least every alternate meal should have optimal protein. This is because protein does more than just 'build muscle'.

We will dive deeper into the 'protein in every alternate meal' concept in a later chapter.

Building the Habit

For now, what are we accomplishing with all this?

Habit formation!

When you eat by the clock, before hunger rises, you are essentially training your body and brain to expect food at regular intervals. Within a few weeks, your hunger cues begin to realign naturally. Your body starts sending signals around the same time each day because it recognises the rhythm.

It is similar to muscle memory, but for your metabolism.

For those who often say 'I just do not feel hungry until late afternoon', this is exactly what they need. Once you start eating at consistent times, your appetite improves, digestion becomes more efficient, and your energy remains stable, avoiding unpredictable peaks and crashes.

And it is this habit that helps you navigate those busier and tougher days. The hunger becomes automatic and no longer requires effort.

Anecdote 8

From boardroom snacks to balanced meals

There was a corporate client of mine working at one of the big four investment banking firms: high pressure, endless meetings, and the kind of stress that makes you forget your own name, let alone your meals.

He was someone who gained weight easily, so his solution was to eat less. Or at least, that is what he believed.

Most days went like this: he would skip breakfast, rush into back-to-back meetings, and survive on coffees, sometimes four… sometimes six. When hunger struck, he would grab whatever the conference room offered: chips, biscuits, *samosas*. At 8:00 p.m., he would drag himself home, convinced 'I barely ate today, I deserve a good dinner', and then overeat before crashing straight into bed.

When he came to me, he was not just struggling with weight; his energy was erratic, his concentration was declining and he felt out of control with food.

So we did not start with a restriction.

We began with a routine.

Breakfast became a non-negotiable part of the day.

We identified realistic food and drink options for him during busy weekdays—choices he could finish between two calls without causing energy spikes or crashes.

Slowly, something shifted.

He noticed he no longer binge-ate on meeting-room snacks. His coffee consumption decreased naturally. His dinners stopped being these massive 'make-up' meals. His energy levels stabilised. And without trying to lose weight, he began losing inches.

Sometimes, the biggest transformation does not come from eating less, but from eating right, consistently, even in a stressful world.

Myths and Truths

1. *Myth:* 'A calorie is a calorie; it does not matter whether you eat it at breakfast or dinner.'

   Truth: Your body does not use calories the same way throughout the day.

   Morning calories are burned more efficiently because insulin sensitivity, cortisol levels, and metabolic rate are higher.

   At night, energy demand drops, and the body shifts towards storage rather than using it. Therefore, timing is important; align your intake with your activity to prevent unnecessary fat storage.

2. *Myth:* 'Small, frequent meals boost your metabolism.'

   Truth: Metabolic rate does not increase just because you eat six times a day. Total calories burned during digestion depend on the amount and type of food, not on how often you eat. Some thrive on two to three meals, while others do better with four to five. There is no one-size-fits-all rule.

3. *Myth:* 'Fasted workouts burn more fat and are better for everyone.'

   Truth: Fasted workouts can make the body rely more on fat for energy during that session. However, using more fat as fuel at the moment does not automatically mean you will lose more overall body fat.[4] Fat loss depends on overall calorie balance across the day and week, since carbohydrates, fats, and even protein can all be used for energy.

   For many women, fuelling correctly during training improves strength, energy, recovery and hormonal balance, ultimately leading to better long-term results.

4. *Myth:* 'If you eat early, you will get hungry again faster.'

   Truth: Hunger is regulated more by hormones than by the clock.

   If breakfast includes protein, fibre, and fat, hunger stabilises, and cravings reduce. If breakfast consists only of carbs, hunger increases, but that depends on the composition, not the timing.

The Takeaway

- Eat four to five times a day. Structure your meals rather than grazing mindlessly.
- Eat on a schedule, not just when you are hungry. It helps reset your metabolism and build consistent eating habits.
- Maintain a three- to four-hour interval between meals, avoiding periods that are too short (to avoid grazing) or too long (to prevent energy dips).

- Count every calorie-containing bite as a meal, because even small bites trigger metabolic changes.
- Include protein in alternate meals; it is essential for recovery, metabolism, and sustained energy.

Your body is a system that thrives on rhythm and discipline. When you feed it consistently and purposefully, it rewards you with better digestion, a stable mood, improved sleep and lasting energy.

So the next time you think of 'eating by the clock', do not see it as rigidity, see it as discipline. Because the more predictable your habits are, the more efficient your body becomes at thriving within them.

To Reiterate

- Meal frequency is flexible: most people do best with four to five structured meals; it is a framework, not a fixed rule.
- Every calorie counts as a meal, as it starts digestion: insulin rises, enzymes activate, and metabolism responds instantly.
- Structure beats grazing.
- Four to six eating occasions spaced across the day support energy and recovery.
- Eating at similar times daily regulates circadian rhythm, cortisol and appetite signals.
- Do not rely only on hunger: stress, long work hours and irregular schedules distort true hunger cues.
- Rhythm builds habit: regular meal timing retrains hunger cues and creates predictable, effortless eating patterns.
- Your body thrives on structure.

A Note from Me to You

Most people do not struggle with food because they lack discipline; they struggle because their eating rhythm is chaotic. Even a single calorie triggers hormonal and digestive responses, and when eating occurs at random times, the body never achieves the stability it needs to manage energy, digestion, recovery, and appetite.

This chapter is meant to help you restore that rhythm. Eating by the clock is not rigidity; it is structure. And once your meals become predictable, your metabolism adjusts accordingly. Your hunger cues reset, your energy stabilises and your body finally starts working with you, not against you.

Habit 6

Start building meal timing

Aim to keep a three- to four-hour gap between meals. This helps maintain steady energy, prevents extreme hunger and keeps your metabolism running smoothly.

Start food logging: record everything you eat and drink. If your hydration habit is already solid, you can skip recording water intake; otherwise, include it, too. The goal is to start noticing the difference between what you think you are doing and what you are actually doing. Often, our assumptions about eating habits do not match reality, and writing things down helps reveal that.

Many successful people in health and fitness swear by food logs. Why? Because tracking your intake helps you naturally identify mistakes and patterns. This allows you to reflect: What went wrong? What can I do differently next time? How can I develop strategies to improve?

Food logging is not about perfection; it is about awareness, learning, and making consistent improvements. Once you develop this habit, establishing structured meal times and healthier eating patterns becomes much easier.

7

Carbohydrates: Friends, Not Foes

In Chapter 6, we discussed meal frequency: how often you should eat, and the importance of timing for your metabolism and hormones.

But frequency alone does not determine the effectiveness of your nutrition.

What truly completes the picture is the composition of those meals. That is why I emphasised the need to ensure there is protein in every other meal, or even better, to include protein in every meal to create a complete meal.

So, what exactly is a complete meal?

A complete meal consists of a balanced combination of three macronutrients:

- Protein is essential for repair and muscle maintenance.
- Fat is important for hormonal health and nutrient absorption.
- Carbohydrates are needed for energy and recovery.

Think of a complete meal as a team effort: each macronutrient has a job, and none works well alone.

These three are the only macronutrients. Vitamins, minerals and antioxidants are classified as micronutrients, which work best when macronutrient intake is well balanced.

Many people focus on minor details while ignoring the bigger picture. Without addressing the overarching concepts, it becomes challenging to resolve the smaller issues.

If the foundation is weak, the details will not fix the structure.

A complete meal is essential for your body as it helps stabilise blood sugar levels, support hormone function and maintain energy throughout the day.

It is important to understand that no food consists solely of one macronutrient. Most foods contain all three macronutrients—carbohydrates, proteins and fats—in varying proportions. The classification of foods into carbohydrate-rich, protein-rich or fat-rich categories is based on the macronutrient that predominates, not on excluding the others.

With this foundation in place, let us take a closer look at the first macronutrient we will explore: carbohydrates, which serve as the body's primary energy source.

Understanding Carbohydrates

The Body's Primary Energy Source

Energy does not come from willpower; it comes from fuel.

Carbohydrates, along with protein and fat, form the foundation of our diet. However, in recent years, carbohydrates have gained an undeserved reputation as dietary villains. With trends promoting low-carb diets and the belief that 'carbs make you fat', many people actively try to eliminate carbohydrates from their meals in pursuit of weight loss, improved metabolic health, or better blood sugar control. What many of these individuals fail to recognise is that fibre is a type of carbohydrate and is often the very nutrient their bodies are desperately lacking.

Some people mistakenly label sugar as toxic, not realising that all digestible carbohydrates—regardless of their source—ultimately contribute to the body's glucose-based energy system.

On average, carbohydrates are the fastest-digesting macronutrient, meaning they are converted into usable energy more quickly than proteins or fats.

Glucose, the simplest form of sugar, is the primary fuel that your body relies on. Whether you eat rice, *roti*, fruit, or bread, your body converts these foods into glucose to fuel your muscles, organs, and brain. In fact, the brain alone uses roughly one-fifth of the body's daily glucose requirements.[1]

This is why sugar is not toxic. The problem lies in chronic excess, poor timing, and lack of metabolic context.

Context changes how the same food behaves in the body.

Think of glucose as the currency your body uses to pay for every function, from blinking your eyes to lifting weights.

Types of Carbohydrates

Complex and Simple

Although all carbohydrates ultimately convert to glucose, they do not behave the same way in the body.

Broadly, carbohydrates can be classified into two categories.

Complex Carbohydrates: The Slow Burners

The difference is not good versus bad; it is speed, structure and amount.

Many people talk about 'cutting carbs', usually referring to grains like rice or wheat. However, they often overlook the fact that grains also provide dietary fibre, a crucial nutrient for digestion, metabolic health, hormonal balance, and long-term disease prevention.

To grasp the importance of fibre, it is essential to look at carbohydrates in a broader context, beyond just calories and blood sugar rise. Complex carbohydrates are particularly rich in fibre.

Complex carbohydrates contain starch and fibre. This structure allows them to be digested more slowly, releasing glucose gradually into the bloodstream.

This slower release helps

- maintain steady energy;
- control hunger; and
- prevent sharp blood sugar spikes and crashes.

Examples of foods that provide a slower release of energy include:

- Whole grains: whole wheat, brown rice, millets, quinoa, oats
- Vegetables: leafy greens, cucumbers, lady fingers, bell peppers
- Roots and tubers: carrots, ginger, sweet potatoes, beets, colocasia

'Slow digestion' does not imply that digestion is sluggish. Rather, it means that digestion occurs at a rate that promotes stable blood sugar and a steady release of insulin.

This steady process allows insulin to do its function effectively, transporting glucose into cells for energy, storing some of it as glycogen in the liver and muscles, and using the rest as needed.

The result is that you feel energetic, satisfied and calm for a longer period.

Now, what is fibre?

Dietary fibre is a type of carbohydrate that cannot be digested or absorbed in the small intestine. Unlike sugars and starches, fibre passes through the digestive tract largely intact. This unique characteristic is precisely what gives fibre its powerful health benefits.

For clarity: while all fibre is a carbohydrate, not all carbohydrates are fibre.

When people cut carbs, they often cut the very thing their gut needs most—fibre.

Dietary fibre is broadly classified into two main types, both of which are essential for optimal health.

1. **Soluble Fibre:** Soluble fibre dissolves in water, creating a gel-like substance in the gut. The process slows down digestion, delays gastric emptying, feeds beneficial gut bacteria and moderates the absorption of glucose and lipids.

Common sources of soluble fibre found in different foods include the following:

- Oats and barley (complex carbs)
- Fruits such as apples, citrus, and berries (simple carbs)
- Legumes like lentils and beans (sources of protein)
- Psyllium husk (a dietary supplement)
- Flaxseeds and chia seeds (sources of healthy fats)

2. **Insoluble Fibre:** Insoluble fibre does not dissolve in water. It adds bulk to the stool and promotes efficient movement of food through the digestive tract. It supports bowel regularity and contributes to gut motility.

Common sources of insoluble fibre include the following:

- Whole wheat and wheat bran (complex carbs)
- Parboiled rice and brown rice (complex carbs)
- Popcorn (complex carbs)
- Nuts and seeds (healthy fats)
- Vegetables such as leafy greens, carrots, and cauliflower (complex carbs)
- Fruits that are eaten with their skin, such as berries, apples and pears (simple carbs)

A healthy diet contains both types, as they work synergistically rather than independently.

Your gut does not need perfection: it needs variety.

Fibre and the Gut Microbiome

One of the most important roles of fibre is its interaction with gut microbiota. Certain fibres, known as fermentable fibres or prebiotics, serve as food for beneficial gut bacteria.

When gut bacteria ferment fibre, they produce short-chain fatty acids (SCFAs).[2] These compounds strengthen the gut lining, reduce intestinal inflammation, improve insulin sensitivity, regulate appetite, and support immune function.

Slower digestion usually means a calmer metabolic response.

A low-fibre diet starves beneficial bacteria, thereby reducing microbial diversity. This reduction is consistently linked to metabolic disorders, obesity, and inflammatory conditions.

Fibre, Blood Sugar and Insulin Response

One of the biggest misconceptions surrounding carbohydrates is that all carbs cause a spike in blood sugar levels. However, fibre fundamentally alters this response.

When carbohydrate-rich foods are high in fibre, glucose absorption occurs more slowly. As a result, blood sugar levels rise gradually, which reduces the demand for insulin.[3]

This is why whole fruits have a different effect on blood sugar compared to fruit juices, and why whole grains behave differently than refined flour, even if their carbohydrate content appears similar on paper.

Most metabolic problems do not appear suddenly; they build quietly over time.

Insulin Sensitivity: The Silent Key to Health

Two people can eat the same meal and yet experience very different blood sugar responses.

Insulin allows glucose to move from the bloodstream into cells for energy, and the body's response varies due to differences in insulin sensitivity.

When insulin sensitivity is high, smaller amounts of insulin can effectively manage blood glucose levels. However, when sensitivity declines, the body requires more insulin to accomplish the same task.

A fibre-rich diet, along with eating pace and meal composition, significantly influences insulin sensitivity. Such dietary patterns help slow the digestion and absorption of carbohydrates, which in turn reduces the sudden demand for insulin.

Changes in insulin sensitivity typically occur gradually and often without clear symptoms, making them easy to overlook. However, insulin sensitivity plays a central role in maintaining long-term metabolic health.

Insulin sensitivity is influenced not only by carbohydrates but also by how we move, eat, sleep, and recover. These topics will be explored later in this book.

Insulin sensitivity also follows the body's circadian rhythm. In many individuals, it tends to be higher earlier in the day and may gradually decline towards the evening, which means the body often handles carbohydrates more efficiently during the morning and daytime hours.

Blood Sugar Rise Versus Spike: What Is Normal and What Is Not

A rise in blood sugar is physiological (normal), not pathological (disease-related).

When carbohydrates are consumed, blood sugar levels increase. This increase is a normal physiological response and is the reason insulin is produced. Insulin helps move glucose from the bloodstream into cells for energy use or storage for later use.

The problem is not simply a rise in blood sugar but rather a spike—a rapid, excessive or prolonged elevation that the body struggles to regulate. Whether a rise remains controlled or escalates into a spike depends on several factors, including portion size, fibre content, meal composition, timing, and insulin sensitivity. It is important to note that carbohydrates themselves do not inherently cause spikes; rather, it is the context in which they are consumed that matters.

Fibre and Weight Regulation

Fibre plays a crucial role in weight management through multiple mechanisms. It enhances satiety by increasing chewing time and promoting gastric distension. It also modulates gut bacteria that are linked to energy extraction.

Fibre does not force weight loss; it makes overeating harder.

A diet rich in protein and fats but chronically low in fibre may initially suppress appetite. However, over time, it can lead to constipation, poor gut health, altered lipid profiles, increased inflammation, reduced dietary diversity and unstable blood glucose regulation that may also affect sleep quality.

Vegetables to Regulate Portion Naturally

This is where vegetables play a crucial role in our meals. Beyond their fibre content, vegetables influence how much we eat, how quickly we eat and how full we feel during a meal.

Vegetables do not just feed the body; they guide how much we eat.

Satiety Signalling and Eating Pace

It takes approximately 20 minutes for the stomach and gut hormones to signal a feeling of fullness to the brain. Raw vegetables require more chewing, which slows down the pace of eating. When a meal begins with raw vegetables or a salad, this slower start effectively 'buys time' for the satiety signals from the gut to reach the brain. As a result, by the time the main meal begins, appetite is already partially regulated. This natural process helps control portion sizes without deliberate restriction.

Do Not Drink Your Fruits and Vegetables

Eating whole vegetables has a digestive advantage over drinking juices or soups. Chewing allows food to mix thoroughly with saliva, which contains salivary amylase—an enzyme that initiates carbohydrate digestion in the mouth.

Whole foods slow us down; liquids let excess slip in unnoticed.

Your body is designed to perform chewing and digestion, so it is best not to outsource these processes to a blender. Liquid foods pass through the mouth more quickly, reducing this important initial digestive interaction. Although nutrient absorption is eventually completed in the intestine, this early step plays a significant role in the speed of digestion, blood glucose response, and satiety.[4]

A Natural Way to Create a Calorie Deficit

Additionally, eating whole foods requires more physical effort for chewing, swallowing, and digestion compared to liquids. As a result, the body uses slightly more energy to process them. While the difference in calories may be modest, the combination of slower eating, improved satiety, and the extra energy expended during digestion can contribute to a small but meaningful calorie deficit without deliberate restriction.

For many people, especially in the first few months of dietary changes, adopting such habits can improve appetite control and support fat loss without the need for calorie counting or deprivation.

Fibre Guidelines and Reality

Most people are not failing at discipline; they are missing optimal fibre.

The general recommendation for adults is 25–30 grams of fibre per day.[5]

However, studies show that the average intake in many populations ranges from 10 to 15 grams per day, which is nearly half of the recommended amount.

This gap is rarely due to a lack of awareness of vegetables, but rather to the fear of carbohydrates, an over-reliance on refined or ultra-processed foods, and an excessive focus on protein at the expense of fibre-rich options.

True carbohydrate wisdom lies not in avoidance, but in discrimination.

Simple Carbohydrates: The Quick Fix

Simple carbohydrates have a simpler structure and are quickly broken down by the body, providing rapid energy—sometimes within minutes to an hour. This quick digestion often occurs because these carbohydrates may lack fibre or contain high levels of natural or added sugar.

Examples of simple carbohydrates include the following:

- Fruits
- White rice, *poha*, puffed rice, semolina, refined flour
- Table sugar
- Coconut sugar, honey, jaggery
- Dates, raisins, dried fruits
- Sweets, desserts, pastries, juices, aerated drinks
- Cookies, cakes, chocolates, and ice creams

Because they are quickly absorbed, they raise blood sugar more quickly.

The Unique Case of Fruits

Fruits are technically simple carbohydrates, but they have a different effect on the body compared to refined sugars.

Fruits contain fructose, which must first be processed by the liver before it can be converted into glucose for energy. Additionally, fruits are also rich in fibre, water and micronutrients, all of which help slow digestion and absorption. This leads to a gentler and more gradual rise in blood sugar levels.

As a result, fruits generally affect blood sugar differently than desserts or refined sugars. However, like all carbohydrate sources, fruits still contribute to total sugar intake. Therefore, it is advisable to be mindful of portion sizes rather than consuming them without limits.

What Counts as Sugar?

Sugar is not limited to just white or refined sugar. Any sugar added during cooking, baking, or processing counts as 'added sugar', even when it comes from sources perceived as 'healthier'.

Honey, jaggery, coconut sugar, dates, maple syrup, and similar ingredients still function as sugars when added to recipes.

Sugar is a treat; do not look for health in it.

While some of these sweeteners may contain small amounts of minerals or antioxidants, they are still concentrated sources of simple carbohydrates that can raise blood glucose and insulin levels. From a metabolic and calorie perspective, the body does not meaningfully distinguish between refined sugar and natural sweeteners once added to food. These foods are not 'free foods' and should be consumed with portion awareness, while keeping within the overall daily sugar budget.

Portion Matters

Simple carbohydrates must certainly be portion-controlled. And do not forget that 'fruits too are still simple carbohydrates'. So they must also be consumed mindfully and with awareness; they also cannot be eaten endlessly throughout the day.

So, what is the portion of fruits?

I generally recommend not eating more than one fruit at a time or a quantity equivalent to one small fruit. For instance, one portion would be: one small apple or banana; half of a small mango, ten to fifteen seedless grapes, or half to one cup of watermelon.

For most people, a practical portion guideline is to have one small fruit per sitting, adjusting based on individual activity levels, metabolic health, and overall carbohydrate intake. It is best to avoid large fruit bowls or fruit juices.

Fruits are easy to overconsume because of their natural sweetness and appealing taste. A common mistake is combining multiple fruits in one serving, assuming that more fruit automatically means better nutrition.

This issue is amplified with smoothies and juices. One glass of fruit juice often contains the sugar equivalent of three or more servings of fruit, and consuming it in liquid form can lead to rapid, excessive sugar intake.

Like all foods, portion size matters. Eating anything in excess can become unhealthy.

> **Portion awareness is not restriction; it is respect for the body's limits.**

A useful practical guideline for many people is to prioritise vegetables over fruits, aiming for roughly three servings of vegetables for every serving of fruit throughout the day.

Added Sugar Guidelines

The World Health Organization recommends limiting added sugars to less than 5–10 per cent of daily calorie intake.[6] In a 1,500-calorie diet, this translates to approximately 80–140 calories or about 4–7 teaspoons of added sugar per day. For better metabolic health, it is advisable to stay closer to the lower end of this range, ideally below 5 per cent, as recommended by the National Institute of Nutrition in India.[7]

> **The body counts sugar by quantity, not by labels.**

This includes sugars from sources such as table sugar, honey, jaggery, syrups, dates, raisins and fruit juices.

Replacing white sugar with honey or dates does not make the food portion-free. While these options may contain small amounts of minerals or antioxidants, they are still sugars and should be counted in the same way, gram for gram.

In practice, I often see people adding twice as much honey or jaggery when replacing sugar, as these alternatives are generally less sweet than sugar. This can lead to a mismatch between intention and outcome. From a metabolic standpoint, consuming half a teaspoon of regular table sugar may be more beneficial than consuming a full teaspoon of honey or jaggery.

The key point is this: anything that counts as added sugar, whether it is white sugar, honey, jaggery, syrups, or dates, should be treated as a treat rather than a source of nutrition. When we start to seek nutrition from treats, it becomes easy and almost unintentional to overconsume.

For this reason, I generally recommend limiting added sugar in beverages to a maximum of one teaspoon per cup, ideally closer to half a teaspoon, and keeping total daily sugar from beverages under two teaspoons.

I Recommend Eating Fruits or Sweets First

Contrary to the traditional belief that sweets should be eaten last, I often recommend having fruits or even a small sweet before a meal or on an empty stomach, rather than after a heavy meal. This can be a good option for those who choose to include sweets in their meals.

Sometimes when you eat matters as much as what you eat.

This discussion is not about encouraging excessive sugar consumption; rather, it is about the importance of digestive sequencing.

How Digestive Sequencing May Help

This recommendation is based on years of real-world observation with clients who struggle with irritable bowel syndrome, bloating, gas, or gut sensitivity. While research on meal sequencing is still evolving, I have observed that some individuals experience less discomfort when they consume fast-digesting carbohydrates earlier in their meals, rather than after heavy mixed meals.

From a digestion standpoint, simple sugars are digested quickly and move rapidly from the stomach into the small intestine.

However, when these sugars are eaten after a large mixed meal, especially one high in fat and protein, overall digestion slows down. In sensitive individuals, this delay can cause some sugars to linger longer in the gut, increasing the likelihood of fermentation and gas production.

Fermentation occurs when unabsorbed carbohydrates reach the bacteria-rich areas of the gut, primarily the colon or prematurely in conditions like SIBO (small intestinal bacterial overgrowth). The bacteria feed on these sugars, producing gases such as hydrogen, methane or sulphur, leading to bloating, discomfort or odorous gas.

This is often why foods like eggs or protein get blamed for digestive discomfort, when the actual issue may stem from delayed sugar digestion.

Fast-digesting carbohydrates are comparable to a Ferrari, while fats and proteins move more slowly, like a heavy truck. When faster-digesting foods are consumed after slower ones, it can lead to congestion in the digestive system. To promote smoother digestion, some people may benefit from eating faster-digesting foods first.

When simple sugars are eaten first, they are more likely to be absorbed earlier in the digestive tract, allowing for the rest of the meal to digest at its natural pace.

For some individuals, consuming fast-digesting foods first and slower foods later may help reduce digestive discomfort.

Digestion works best when foods move at their natural pace.

There is also a behavioural and satiety advantage.

Eating whole fruit before a meal can improve fullness and reduce total calorie intake.[8] Additionally, it has psychological benefits: when people are aware they have already eaten fruit or a dessert, they tend to portion the main meal more mindfully.

In contrast, when dessert is eaten at the end of the meal, most people do not monitor their portion sizes for the main course and often 'make space' for dessert. This habit can result in overeating and exceeding calorie limits.

Impact on Blood Sugar

Many people believe that eating fruit or dessert at the end of a meal prevents a spike in blood sugar. However, what is often overlooked is the duration of elevated blood glucose levels. When sugar is consumed after a large mixed meal, especially one high in fat, gastric emptying slows down. This means that glucose absorption happens over a longer period, which can prolong mild increases in glucose levels, even if the peak is lower.

In contrast, when fruit or a small sweet is eaten first, blood glucose may rise more quickly. However, the subsequent intake of protein, fat, and fibre can help stabilise these levels, support insulin function, and reduce the likelihood of a sharp drop in blood sugar levels.

In metabolically healthy individuals, blood glucose typically returns to baseline within about two hours. Thus, the goal is not just to avoid sharp peaks but also to prevent prolonged elevation, both of which are important for maintaining metabolic health.

For individuals with diabetes or significant glucose dysregulation, the overall carbohydrate quantity, their spacing and medical guidance take precedence over the order in which foods are consumed. The question of whether to eat fruit or dessert before or after a meal becomes irrelevant, because simple carbohydrates should ideally not be combined with main meals. In such cases, it is better to consume fruits, sweets, or other simple carbohydrates as separate, planned snacks, rather than alongside a full mixed meal. This approach is not merely about meal sequencing; it is a fundamental dietary principle for managing blood sugar levels. For diabetics, timing, spacing, and portion control are more important than the order in which foods are eaten.

Who Benefits Most from This Approach

This approach appears particularly helpful for the following groups:

- Individuals with IBS, bloating or gas
- Those who feel heavy or uncomfortable after meals
- People with sensitive or reactive digestive systems
- Individuals with a genetic predisposition, who notice improved carbohydrate tolerance with strategic timing

Many clients report experiencing reduced bloating, improved appetite regulation, and better overall comfort.

Timing Simple Carbohydrates Wisely

Simple carbohydrates should be used strategically, when your body actually benefits from that quick energy.

There are two times when simple carbohydrates work especially well for the body:

- *Upon waking up:* After an overnight fast, cortisol levels tend to be higher in the morning due to the dawn phenomenon. Consuming a small, quick source of energy, such as fruit, can help ease the transition from a fasted state to a fed state and stabilise energy levels. This is why many people find that starting their day with fruit before breakfast works well for them.
- *After physical activity:* Exercise increases insulin sensitivity and depletes glycogen stores.[9] Consuming a simple carbohydrate post-workout helps replenish energy and supports recovery. This creates a more forgiving metabolic window, allowing room for a small dessert if desired.

Many of my clients find this a helpful strategy to enjoy their favourite sweet without feeling deprived or as though they are 'on a diet'. This approach helps them stay consistent and adhere to their goals better.

However, it is important not to assume you can indulge in sweets without limits. The goal is to avoid deprivation, which can lead to bingeing later on. Hence, portion control is essential.

Anecdote 9

The end of the 'chotu sa *bite' habit*

A thirty-eight-year-old woman once came to me seeking help with weight loss. When I reviewed her food logs, a clear pattern emerged.

She had small portions of *mithai* sprinkled throughout the day: 'just one small bite', '*chotu sa* bite', 'only about a teaspoon of cake'.

These tiny bites occurred four to five times a day, and each time she reassured herself that it was too little to matter.

When we started working together, I offered her a very different suggestion. I told her she could enjoy one full sweet of her choice, guilt-free, after her workout, but advised her to refrain from eating sweets for the rest of the day.

She looked at me in disbelief.

'Are you serious? I can eat one sweet every day if I exercise?'

When I nodded in agreement, she visibly relaxed.

'That is easy,' she said. 'I exercise anyway.'

She was concerned, of course, about sugar spikes, weight gain, and whether this would undo all her effort. Once I explained the logic behind it, she agreed to give it a try.

Post-workout, she started savouring her sweets slowly and actually enjoying them.

Her trainer found it amusing and joked that she was wasting her workout efforts. She just smiled and kept enjoying her treat.

Five days later, she messaged me. 'Mitushi, this is shocking,' she wrote. 'I do not even feel like eating *mithai* through the day anymore.'

Having one proper portion without any fear made her feel truly satisfied.

There was no fear, no guilt, and no feeling of deprivation—only pure joy.

Two months later, she went on a holiday. By then, her fat loss was consistent and sustainable.

When she returned, she shared something that stayed with me: 'This is the first holiday where I did not stress about food at all.

I ate to nourish myself, moved more, had dessert when I wanted, and enjoyed it.'

She had not gained weight. In fact, when she measured herself, she had lost half an inch off her waist during the holiday.

That, to me, is the real success: not control through fear, but freedom through understanding.

Satisfaction ends grazing; fear keeps it alive.

Effects of Simple Carbohydrates in Excess

Now imagine eating a large quantity of white rice, bread, dessert, or any other simple carbohydrate that is quickly digested, especially when you are not physically active.

The glucose from this food or meal quickly enters your bloodstream, causing your blood sugar levels to spike. In response, your body releases insulin to help lower excess glucose in your bloodstream, as elevated blood sugar levels are physiologically not healthy.

Insulin effectively clears sugar from the bloodstream, but it can sometimes overcompensate.

As a result, your blood sugar may drop too quickly, leaving you with an energy slump. During this period, you might experience the following:

- Increased hunger (even if you just ate)
- Irritable or low energy
- Craving for something sweet or starchy

It is not the carbohydrate; it is the mismatch between fuel and demand.

For individuals with lower insulin sensitivity or lower energy needs at that moment, this rapid increase in blood sugar can be followed by an equally rapid decrease. This cycle can lead to hunger, fatigue, and cravings. Over time, this pattern increases the likelihood of fat storage.

This is why portion size, timing, and activity level matter when considering simple carbohydrates.

A Note for Diabetics

If you are diabetic or insulin-resistant, you can still apply some of these principles, but you need to pay closer attention to quantity, timing, food pairings, and seek professional guidance.

A well-managed diabetic may be able to tolerate half a serving of a low-GI fruit (such as apple, guava, papaya, or orange) in the morning, and this should always be followed by some protein or fat.

Desserts or *mithai* should only be considered after physical activity and in very small portions.

Anyone with poorly controlled blood sugar or an elevated HbA1c should avoid self-experimentation and consult a qualified nutrition professional or their treating physician or endocrinologist.

Understanding Glycaemic Index and Glycaemic Load

The glycaemic index (GI) is a scale that ranks carbohydrate-containing foods based on how quickly they raise blood sugar levels after consumption. The slower a food raises your blood sugar, the better it is for maintaining steady energy and preventing crashes.

However, looking at GI alone does not provide the complete picture. That is where glycaemic load (GL) comes in. GL takes into account both the quality (GI) and the quantity (portion) of a food.[10]

This is where many well-intentioned substitutions go wrong. I often see traditional sweets like *laddoo*s or *halwa* prepared with sweeteners such as stevia, monk fruit, dates, or jaggery, and mistakenly assumed to be low impact. While these sweeteners may contribute little to blood sugar rise, the overall GL of the dish is still determined by the total amount of carbohydrates present, which include flours, grains, nuts, dried fruits, and portion sizes.

In many cases, the majority of calories in sweets come not from sugar, but from fats and other ingredients. When sugar is replaced with 'healthier' alternatives, people often feel justified in eating larger portions, which increases both calorie intake and GL. In this context, it is not the sweetness that matters; it is the combination, quantity, and frequency of consumption that determine the metabolic impact.

In real life, GL matters more because we rarely eat foods in isolation or in their pure form. We usually eat meals that include carbohydrates, proteins, and fats. This combination affects how the body processes glucose.

Carbohydrates Must Not Be Feared

Carbohydrates remain the body's primary dietary source of glucose, especially for the brain, active muscles, and red blood cells.

In fact, your brain alone accounts for roughly one-fifth of your total glucose consumption at rest.

However, at some point, the term 'low-carb' became a synonym for 'healthy'. In reality, carbohydrates are not the enemy; they are essential for physical energy, mental clarity, hormone production, and digestive health.

Now you also know that fibre is a carbohydrate and plays a crucial role in keeping the gut healthy, feeding your gut microbiome, controlling blood sugar, slowing digestion, and keeping you full for longer. If you remove carbs or grains from your diet, it means removing fibre, which can lead to poor gut health. A healthy body cannot be achieved without a healthy gut.

So, do not fear carbs; learn to use them wisely.

Your body thrives on discipline, not restriction. By eating carbs smartly, you can enjoy stable energy levels, better workouts, improved sleep, and sharper focus.

When viewed in this context, carbohydrates transition from being something to fear to something to understand and use intentionally.

Carbohydrates are not the villains of your story; they are the fuel that powers you.

Myths and Truths

1. *Myth:* 'Carbohydrates make you fat.'

   Truth: Excess calories, not carbohydrates alone, lead to weight gain. Carbs support energy, recovery, and metabolic health when eaten in appropriate portions, aligned with activity levels, and combined with protein and fat.

The body's goal is not elimination but adaptation.

2. *Myth:* 'All carbs spike blood sugar.'

   Truth: The blood sugar response is influenced by fibre content, food form, portion size, meal composition, and insulin sensitivity; not just the presence of carbohydrates.

3. *Myth:* 'Cutting carbs is the fastest way to improve health.'
   Truth: Many people see initial improvements due to decreased calorie intake and the avoidance of ultra-processed foods, not because carbohydrates are inherently harmful. Long-term carb elimination often reduces fibre intake and negatively affects gut health.
4. *Myth:* '"Healthy sugars" do not count.'
   Truth: Honey, jaggery, coconut sugar, dates, and syrups are still sugars when added to food. The body reacts to the total amount consumed, rather than the type of sugar or its source.
5. *Myth:* 'Carbohydrates are optional.'
   Truth: Carbohydrates are the body's primary dietary source of glucose, essential for brain function, physical performance, recovery, and fibre intake. Avoiding them is not a sign of intelligence.
6. *Myth:* 'Carbohydrates cause blood sugar spikes.'
   Truth: Not every 'rise' in blood sugar is a 'spike'. Gradual rises are part of normal physiology; sharp or prolonged elevations are the concern.
7. *Myth:* 'Eating carbohydrates at night causes weight gain.'
   Truth: Weight gain is primarily driven by total energy intake and metabolic context rather than the time of day. Carbohydrates eaten at night can still be beneficial for recovery and glycogen replenishment when eaten in appropriate portions and combined with adequate activity. In fact, including carbohydrates at dinner may promote better sleep by helping the body relax and wind down.

8. *Myth:* 'Juicing fruits and vegetables is equivalent to eating them.'
   Truth: Liquid forms bypass chewing, slow digestion speed, and make overconsumption easy. Whole foods are more effective at regulating appetite than their liquid counterparts.
9. *Myth:* 'Low-carb diet automatically means low sugar.'
   Truth: Many low-carb diets often contain high amounts of sugars from fruits, dates, honey, and snacks, which are frequently consumed without awareness of portion sizes.
10. *Myth:* 'If a food is "whole" or "natural", portion does not matter.'
    Truth: Whole foods can still be overconsumed. Health outcomes depend on total intake, digestion speed, and context, not just food quality.
11. *Myth:* 'Sugar is toxic.'
    Truth: Sugar, composed of glucose and fructose, serves as a normal and usable fuel for the body. Problems arise from chronic excess and poor context, rather than from sugar itself. The body's goal is adaptation, not elimination; fear surrounding sugar comes from excessive intake, not its mere presence.

To Reiterate

- A complete meal includes protein, fat, and carbohydrates working together.
- Portion control and timing matter, not labelling them as 'superfood' or 'toxic'.
- Carbohydrates are the primary energy source for the body. They are not the enemy; type and portion determine their impact.

- Carbohydrates are essential for gut health and metabolic rhythm.
- Sugar is not as toxic as it is made out to be. Portion and timing matter.
- Complex carbohydrates support stable energy and blood sugar.
- Simple carbohydrates digest quickly and work best when timed strategically.
- Fruits behave differently from refined sugars due to fibre and lower GL.
- Eating fruits or sweets before meals may help people with sensitive digestion or gut sensitivity.
- Eating vegetables first helps in natural portion control.
- Eating slowly helps control portions and improve satiety.
- Do not drink your fruits and vegetables.

A Note from Me to You

Carbohydrates, including sugar, were never meant to cause harm. This chapter serves as a reminder that the body thrives on balance rather than restriction. When you understand how carbohydrates work, what options to choose, how much to eat, and when to eat them, you stop fighting your body and start working in harmony with it. Instead of eliminating foods, learn to incorporate them wisely. Nourish yourself with intention rather than guilt. Your energy, digestion, and hormones respond best to discipline and consistency. Over the years, I have seen many people report reduced sugar cravings once the fear around sugar is removed. By eating sugar strategically and mindfully, they manage to avoid overconsumption. Even a daily *mithai* can fit into a balanced diet without ill effects when portion sizes are controlled and timing is considered. No deprivation, no guilt. This approach has been my most effective tool for helping people build sustainable eating habits, without waiting for an end date.

Habit 7

Start your meals with vegetables

Start your main meals with vegetables: lunch and dinner.

Aim for a generous serving, prepared as simply as possible. Raw vegetables of your choice, like cucumber, radish, carrot, bell pepper, tomato and lettuce, work better if you can tolerate them. Try to cut these vegetables minimally. A good option is to cut them lengthwise to retain more water and volume; avoid slicing or dicing.

There is no need for heavy dressings; a pinch of salt, basic seasoning, or a squeeze of lime is enough if you prefer.

If raw vegetables do not suit you, choose lightly cooked, sautéed, or grilled vegetables made with minimal oil. Opt for those vegetables that suit you.

Eat your meal slowly and mindfully. Try to take at least 30 minutes to finish your main meals.

This one habit encourages better portion awareness, steadier energy, and more comfortable eating, without changing what you eat, only how you eat.

Track Your Progress

Pause. Reflect. Revisit.

You have now completed seven chapters. Before moving ahead, this is a good moment to pause and check in with yourself.

Go back to the 'Track Your Progress' section from Chapter 3. Take a few minutes to record the same markers again and compare them with your starting point. This is not about judgement or perfection; it is about awareness.

Progress in nutrition is often subtle. It shows up in how you feel, how you function, and how your body responds over time. Revisiting these markers helps you notice those shifts and keeps the process grounded in your own experience.

This step puts the responsibility where it belongs—with you.

Track these again.

Daily measurements

- Water intake: ______ litres per day
- Sleep duration: ______ hours per day
- Sleep quality: Poor/Good/Excellent
- Energy levels throughout the day: Poor/Good/Excellent

Weekly assessments

- Sugar cravings: High/Moderate/None
- Hunger pangs/craving for snacks: Often/Moderate/Rarely
- Bowel movement: Regular/Constipation/Frequent indigestion
- Flatulence/gas/acidity/heartburn: Severe/Moderate/Rarely

8

Proteins: Your Body's Building Blocks

THIS IS ONE OF the most important topics to understand. Take the time to read it, revisit it, and let the ideas really sink in so they can quietly guide your choices every time you eat.

In the earlier chapters, I shared a simple yet powerful insight about protein: 'Manage your protein through the day. Every alternate meal must have protein, or it should be a complete meal.'

Now, let us break down the reasons behind this advice.

Have you ever noticed how people casually mention joint pain, such as back pain, knee pain, shoulder stiffness, or that persistent neck tension? These aches are so common that we have almost accepted them as a normal part of ageing or as a side effect.

However, in many cases, these pains indicate something deeper: the gradual loss of muscle mass, which can exacerbate issues like cartilage wear or connective tissue stress.

While muscle building is a separate subject, it is important to note that protein provides the raw material needed for muscle repair and helps limit muscle loss when energy intake and training are adequate.

Muscles are more than just making you look fit. They support your joints, stabilise your spine, protect your bones, and allow for easier movement.[1] And it is the protein that builds and maintains these muscles.

In simple terms, protein is an essential nutrient that your body cannot replace with anything else.

We all know that when we eat more food than we need, we tend to gain fat. This applies to carbohydrates, fats, and protein, as surplus calories can be stored as body fat.

Have you ever considered why excess calories are stored as fat instead of muscle? There is much more to this phenomenon than it seems.

In this chapter, we will unravel the true nature of protein, explore how it functions in your body, and explain why getting your protein intake right can completely transform how you feel, perform, and recover.

Why Protein Matters More Than You Think

When most people hear the word 'protein', they immediately think of muscles. While muscles are part of the story, they are far from the whole picture. Proteins are present in every cell of your body. They both building blocks and builders. They provide structure, acting as the bricks, while also functioning as the construction workers that repair, replace, and renew tissues.

So, while carbohydrates and fats fuel your daily activities, protein fuels your body's renewal processes.

Consider this: we often worry about energy, but what about repair?

What about the parts of you that constantly need rebuilding, such as your skin, hair, nails, and even your immune system?

So, let us take a closer look at proteins.

What Are Proteins Made Of

When people think about protein, they often focus solely on the 'total grams per day'. While this is important, what is frequently overlooked is how the body actually utilises that protein. Not all protein goes directly to muscle, and not all proteins are created equal. Factors such as timing, quality, and completeness matter.

Proteins are composed of smaller units known as amino acids, which are often referred to as the building blocks of life. The body uses about twenty different amino acids. Among these, nine are essential amino acids, meaning that your body cannot produce them on its own, so you must obtain them through your diet.

The remaining amino acids are non-essential, meaning your body can synthesise them as long as it receives the essential ones first.

This highlights that the quality of your protein is as important as the quantity.

Quality of Proteins

The quality of protein refers to the number of amino acids present in protein foods. Based on this, protein foods are classified as complete and incomplete.

Complete Proteins

Complete proteins are considered to be superior proteins, as they contain all nine essential amino acids in the right proportions that your body needs.

- All animal-based proteins—eggs, dairy, meat, fish, and poultry—are complete proteins.

- Among plant-based proteins—soy and its products, including edamame, tofu, tempeh, soy milk—are among the few that qualify as complete proteins.

Why does completeness matter?

If any essential amino acid is present in low amounts, muscle protein synthesis slows down, making the process less efficient. It is similar to trying to build a wall with bricks but having almost no cement to hold them together.

That is why completeness is important: your body needs all nine essential amino acids at once to effectively repair tissues, build muscle, and support functions such as hormone and enzyme production. The body cannot 'partially' complete muscle repair or protein synthesis; it needs the entire set of amino acids to do the job efficiently.

Without this completeness, protein intake may seem adequate, but its actual impact inside the body is compromised.

Incomplete Proteins

Proteins that are missing one or more amino acids are called incomplete proteins. Most plant-based proteins, except soy products, have an incomplete essential amino acid profile. This means that they need to be combined strategically to meet amino acid requirements.[2] Examples of incomplete protein sources include pulses (such as *dal*s, lentils, beans, peas) and gram flour (*besan*).

Pulses like lentils are low in methionine, making it the limiting amino acid in lentils.

Now, the beauty of nature is that it supplies these limiting amino acids in abundance in grains, which our traditional diets have instinctively combined to create complete foods.[3]

This does not mean you need to count amino acids. Traditional food combinations are already balanced; chasing a single nutrient often disrupts the balance.

Grains such as rice, wheat, and millets are higher in carbohydrates, but they also contain some amino acids. While they are low in lysine, they have a good amount of methionine, the limiting amino acid in lentils. Thus, when you combine lentils with another grain, you achieve a complete protein with all the required amino acids.

Consider combinations like *dal* with rice, *dal* with *roti*, *sambar* with *idli*, hummus with pita, and *rajma* with *chawal* or *khichdi*. These combinations balance out the missing amino acids and create a complete protein profile.

So, if you are a vegetarian or vegan, you do not need to worry. Just focus on combining your foods thoughtfully and cooking intelligently.

Time Taken to Digest Protein

Protein digestion begins in the stomach and continues in the small intestine. Depending on the food source and meal composition, the digestion and absorption of most proteins can take anywhere from 2 to 8 hours.

Whey protein is digested and absorbed relatively quickly compared to whole foods, with amino acids entering the bloodstream early on. However, digestion and absorption continue over several hours.[4]

> *Note:* Foods like quinoa, *sattu* and amaranth are primarily carbohydrate sources and provide moderate amounts of protein. They do not contain enough protein to be considered as primary protein sources.
>
> Similarly, nuts, seeds, and peanuts are high in fat and provide some protein, but they are not effective for meeting high-protein targets because of their high calorie density.
>
> So, it is important not to rely on these foods to achieve your daily protein target. They can add a small amount of protein, similar to how rice or wheat flour does, but they should not be your main source of protein.

Cooking, soaking, sprouting and fermenting plant foods significantly improve their digestibility. For example, *dal* soaked overnight or *idli* batter fermented for hours are not just traditional practices; they are grounded in science.

Protein In Your Body

Unlike carbohydrates, which are stored as glycogen, and fats, which are stored in adipose tissue, protein does not have a dedicated storage form in the body. Instead, skeletal muscle serves as the largest functional reserve of amino acids, alongside proteins found in organs and the circulation.[5]

Your body is continuously breaking down muscle tissue, a process known as muscle protein breakdown (MPB) or muscle catabolism.

At the same time, your body is rebuilding these muscle tissues through an ongoing renewal process referred to as muscle protein synthesis (MPS) or muscle anabolism.[6]

Your muscle mass depends on the balance:

If MPS > MPB, you build or maintain muscle.

If MPB > MPS, you lose muscle.

So, MPS is how your body repairs old muscle proteins and builds new ones.

Here is the important part: MPS is 'always' happening, even when you are resting or fasting. The key question is how much MPS is happening and whether it is enough to offset the breakdown?

You do not need to remember these terms. Just remember this: your muscles are constantly being broken down and rebuilt, and what you eat and how you move decide which side wins.

The rate of MPS is heavily dependent on what you eat, when you eat, and how much you move.

Now, when you consume protein-rich foods, they are digested and broken down into finer units called amino acids. These amino acids enter your bloodstream and serve as both raw materials and signals to your body, indicating that it should 'repair and rebuild now'. As a result, MPS rises for a few hours after a protein-containing meal, then gradually returns to baseline levels.

This leads to an important distinction: protein directly stimulates muscle protein synthesis through amino acids, while carbohydrates help reduce muscle protein breakdown by providing energy and promoting insulin-mediated responses. Fats contribute indirectly by supporting energy balance, allowing protein to be spared from being used as fuel.[7]

But there is a catch: MPS is not unlimited.

There is a limit to how much protein can effectively stimulate muscle protein synthesis at one time, often referred to as the ceiling effect of protein. This threshold

That is why protein cannot be replaced by carbs or fats; its role is unique. But it also cannot work well without them.

is based on factors such as age, training status, meal composition, and energy balance.

Your body can only use a limited amount of protein at a time to maximally stimulate muscle repair. Once you exceed this amount, additional protein does not further increase muscle protein synthesis.[8] Instead, that extra protein is used for other functions, such as enzyme production or energy, rather than contributing to additional muscle building. Of course, it can be stored as additional body fat.

Eating more protein is not wrong; it is just not more effective if it is all crammed into one meal.

When protein is used for energy instead of carbohydrates or fats, I refer to it as 'expensive energy'. This is because you are essentially using your body's premium building material—like bricks from your house—to fuel your energy needs, something that carbohydrates and fats can do much more efficiently.

This is where timing and distribution become important. After consuming a high-protein meal, essential amino acids enter the bloodstream and stimulate MPS. MPS rises transiently for a few hours before returning to baseline levels, typically within ~2–4 hours.

By consuming a protein-rich meal every few hours, you create multiple opportunities for MPS to rise.

Spreading protein throughout the day, rather than consuming it all at once, leads to better muscle maintenance and recovery.

Additionally, resistance training enhances this process. When protein consumption is paired with training, MPS increases, leading to the development of more muscle tissue, a topic covered in the chapter on movement. Refer to the table below:

Situation	MPS	MPB	Outcome
Adequate protein + training	High	Controlled	Muscle gain
Adequate protein, no training	Moderate	Controlled	Muscle maintenance
Low protein intake	Low	Higher	Muscle loss
Calorie deficit + low protein	Very low	High	Accelerated muscle loss

Table 8.1: *Protein intake, training, and their effect on muscle gain or loss*

The Car Analogy: Protein Timing and Completeness

Think of muscle building like running an assembly line to build cars.

***Scenario 1* (100 grams protein at once)**

You deliver a truck with 100 car parts to the factory. The workers only have time and space to build one car with thirty parts. So, the other seventy parts are taken away to build roads, power plants, or burned as fuel. They never come back to the car factory.

***Scenario 2* (Incomplete protein, like *dal* alone)**

You deliver most of the car parts, but one essential part is missing. The factory cannot operate at full capacity during that shift, so fewer cars are produced in the available time. If the missing part arrives much later, it may be used in the next production run, but it cannot fully compensate for the lost productivity of the current one.

Both situations reveal the same truth: protein timing and protein quality are just as important as total intake. If you distribute protein evenly across the day and ensure meals include complete proteins or smart combinations like *dal* with rice, *roti*, or yoghurt, your muscles receive a steady, balanced supply of all the components they need, exactly when they need them.

Tip: To promote continuous repair and maintenance in the body throughout the day, it is important to include a quality protein source in every alternate meal, especially if you eat five to six meals daily. Keeping protein in all meals is even more beneficial, as it can be challenging to meet your total daily protein requirement with just two to three meals.

The Protein–Hormone Connection

In practical terms, this simply means spreading protein across meals and not relying on a single large serving to do all the work.

Many key hormones and signalling molecules, including insulin and several neurotransmitters such as dopamine and serotonin, are derived from amino acids.

Protein Builds Muscles, Insulin Protects Them

Many people believe that insulin is only triggered by carbohydrates, but that is not true. Protein can also stimulate insulin release.

So, what does insulin do here?

Amino acids = builders (they add new bricks to your muscle).

Insulin = a security guard (it protects the bricks already in place).

Insulin does not directly build muscle, but it plays a permissive role by reducing muscle protein breakdown and supporting an environment that promotes muscle repair.[9]

Think of insulin as support, not the star of the show. Protein does the building; insulin simply helps protect the progress.

Together, these elements create the perfect environment for your muscles to recover and grow. A well-balanced protein intake supports better energy, mood, and metabolism.

For women, particularly during perimenopause and menopause, maintaining sufficient protein intake can help preserve lean muscle mass, support thyroid health, and stabilise blood sugar levels.

Anecdote 10

A case of misused protein

I would like to return to the same client I mentioned in Anecdote 7.

She had worked with multiple dietitians and nutritionists over the years, yet her hypothyroid symptoms never improved. Her recovery was consistently poor, and even light workouts left her extremely sore for days. Over time, she began blaming her trainers for pushing her 'too hard' and frequently quit, convinced that exercise itself was the problem.

The problem was not the intensity of her training.

She had been put on a zero-grain, salt-free diet for extended periods. With no carbohydrates entering her body, the body had no choice but to burn protein for energy. As a result, the very protein that was supposed to repair her muscles was being used for energy instead, leaving her muscles under-recovered and constantly sore.

However, when we reintroduced carbohydrates, including morning fruits and whole grains, something remarkable happened.

Within a week, her soreness completely disappeared, even though she was now lifting three times the weight she had been lifting earlier.

Her protein intake was similar.

The difference lay in her carbohydrate consumption.

Protein was not contributing to her muscle growth; instead, it was being used up as 'expensive energy'.

This experience reinforced a critical lesson: protein builds muscle, but insulin plays a crucial role in preserving it.

Without sufficient energy intake, even the best protein plan can be counterproductive.

The Thermic Effect of Protein

A Fun Fact

Your body uses energy to digest, absorb and process the food you eat. This is known as the thermic effect of food (TEF).[10]

This does not mean protein magically boosts metabolism, it just means your body works a little harder to process it.

Among the macronutrients, protein has the highest thermic effect, typically ranging from about 20–30 per cent, followed by carbohydrates at roughly 5–15 per cent and fats at around 0–3 per cent. However, these values vary based on food type, processing, and meal composition.

This means eating protein not only builds muscle but also slightly boosts metabolism. This is one reason why high-protein diets are often effective for fat loss. However, if a high-protein diet is poorly planned, it may end up low in fibre, leading to digestive discomfort.

Hence, a balanced diet helps keep the muscles strong, the gut healthy and inflammation low.

Protein and Satiety: Why It Keeps You Full

Protein is the most satiating macronutrient, helping control hunger and reduce cravings. It digests slowly, keeping you full for longer periods, so you do not feel hungry often. Consuming protein increases satiety and can help moderate blood sugar responses when paired with carbohydrates, as it slows digestion and minimises rapid glucose spikes.

If you often feel hungry between meals or find yourself reaching for snacks, check your protein distribution rather than questioning your willpower.

> **If you have ever felt less hungry and more in control after a protein-rich meal, this is why.**

How Much Protein Do You Really Need?

This is one of the most common questions.

The official RDA (Recommended Dietary Allowance) of 0.8 g/kg represents the minimum intake required to prevent deficiency at a population level, not the intake needed to optimise muscle health or performance. In this sense, you may say it is enough to survive, but not to thrive.[11]

For anyone who is active, training, or simply looking to maintain lean muscle mass as they age, a more realistic range is 1.2–1.6 g/kg of body weight.

So, for someone weighing 60 kg, that would translate to approximately 72–96 gm/day, spread across meals.

> **This is not about fear or deficiency; it is about aligning intake with how you live, move and age.**

However, it is important to remember that it is not just about the total amount of protein; the distribution throughout the day also matters.

A simple thumb rule: include 20–30 gm of protein in every main meal and 8–15 gm in your snacks.

How to Assess the Quality of a Protein Source

Not all foods labelled as 'high protein' are actually good sources of protein. This is especially true for packaged foods and protein bars.

So, how can you determine if a food is truly rich in protein or just capitalising on marketing?

There is a very simple way to assess protein quality: divide the total calories of the food by the grams of protein it provides.

Let us take an example.

Imagine a protein bar that claims to be healthy and has the following nutrition profile (as shown in Figure 8.1).

Nutrition Information
Serving Size: 1 bar (45 g)

Nutrient	Per Bar
Energy	**166 kcal**
Protein	**8 g**
Carbohydrates	**20 g**
– Sugars	11 g
– Dietary Fibre	4 g
Total Fat	**6 g**
– Saturated Fat	2.5 g
Sodium	120 mg

Table 8.2: *Example of nutritional information*

You need to take the calories (energy) and divide them by the amount of protein in it.

Energy: 166 kcal

Protein: 8 gm

Now divide:

166 ÷ 8 = 20.75

This means that to obtain 1 gm of protein, you would need to consume over 20 calories.

This is not an efficient way to get protein.

Pure protein provides only 4 calories/gm. Therefore, if a food requires you to consume significantly more calories to acquire each gram of protein, it is likely that most of its energy comes from fats and carbohydrates rather than protein.

While this does not automatically make such foods unhealthy, it does mean they are not efficient sources of protein and should not be counted as lean proteins when trying to meet daily protein requirements. Many packaged foods and protein bars add protein for marketing purposes, but the bulk of their calories often come from sugars or fats.

This calorie-to-protein ratio is therefore a useful screening tool, especially when evaluating protein supplements and packaged products that claim to be 'high protein'. This ratio helps distinguish foods that genuinely provide protein from those that are simply marketed as protein.

Whole foods, however, naturally contain a mix of macronutrients and should not be judged by this ratio alone. Instead, their overall nutritional value, digestibility, micronutrient content, and role in a balanced diet should be considered.

Foods like eggs, dairy products, legumes, tofu, fish and meats may not always score as 'lean' by numbers, but they provide satiety, essential nutrients, and sustained nourishment that isolated metrics cannot capture.

The goal, therefore, is not simply to chase the highest protein number or the lowest calorie ratio, but to choose appropriate protein sources in the right context. This means balancing efficiency with overall diet quality. Once you understand this distinction, meeting your daily protein needs becomes far more practical and sustainable.

So, the next time you pick up a packaged product that claims to be high in protein, do not just read the front label.

Turn it over.

Do the math.

Because when it comes to protein, the quality is just as important as the quantity.

Now that you understand the 'why', let us focus on the 'how' without overthinking it.

Practical Ways to Meet Your Protein Target

Keep in mind that increasing protein intake too quickly can lead to digestive issues. So, it is important to gradually increase your protein consumption, for example, by adding 10–15 gm per day each week. You should also increase your water intake, as more protein requires more water. Monitor your daily bowel movements; as your body adapts and your bowel movements remain regular, you can further increase your protein intake by an additional 10–15 gm if you are not meeting your daily requirements.

- Aim to consume at least 1.2 g/kg body weight of protein daily. Later, it should be adjusted to 1.2–2 g/kg based on your activity level.
- Distribute your total protein intake across three to five meals.
- Combine plant proteins smartly with grains or other complete sources if you are a vegetarian.
- Choose high-quality sources—the leaner, the better—and minimise processed and high-fat foods.
- Do not hesitate to use supplements; use them strategically as needed. But remember, prioritise real food first.

Make sure to include at least one item from the following for each meal or snack, based on your food habits.

Vegan	Vegetarian	Eggetarian	Non-vegetarian
Lentils, beans, chickpeas, peas, sprouts, gram flour + Soy products: edamame, tofu, tempeh, soy milk + Not protein-dense, but may contribute: nuts, seeds, quinoa, amaranth + Plant protein supplement	Dairy products: milk, *paneer*, curd, Greek yoghurt + Whey and casein protein supplements + Vegan options	Eggs + Vegetarian options	Animal sources: chicken, meat, fish, seafood + Eggetarian options

Table 8.3: *Protein sources for vegan, vegetarian, eggetarian and non-vegetarian diets*

Myths and Truths

1. *Myth:* 'Too much protein damages your kidneys.'

   Truth: In healthy individuals, higher protein intake has not been shown to harm kidney function. Adequate hydration supports overall kidney health, though it is not the only factor.
2. *Myth:* 'Plant proteins are incomplete, so they're useless.'

   Truth: Plant proteins are not useless. They just need to be paired intelligently. Indian and Asian diets already contain complementary proteins. A point in favour of plant proteins is that they contain fibre, which animal proteins lack.
3. *Myth:* 'Protein shakes are unnatural.'

   Truth: A protein supplement is simply a concentrated source of clean protein. It is convenient but not mandatory. Use it when food alone does not meet your needs.
4. *Myth:* 'More protein means more muscle.'

   Truth: Building muscle requires a training stimulus. Protein supports the process but does not replace the effort.
5. *Myth:* 'Quinoa is a complete protein source.'

   Truth: Quinoa contains all nine essential amino acids, but it is still a carbohydrate source due to its higher carb ratio. In fact, it has only 1 gram more protein than wheat flour. So, if you use quinoa to meet your protein needs, you may end up consuming more calories than you need.
6. *Myth:* 'Peanuts and peanut butter are good protein sources.'

   Truth: While peanuts and peanut butter contain some protein, they are primarily fat-dense foods, not high-quality protein sources. Most of their calories come from fats, and the protein per calorie is relatively low. They also lack a complete essential amino acid profile, making them better classified as healthy fat sources with some protein rather than true protein foods.

To Reiterate

- Proteins are the fundamental building blocks of the body, and effective repair and growth require the presence of all essential amino acids in adequate amounts.
- MPS increases when amino acids enter the bloodstream; however, there is a limit to this effect—consuming more protein in a single meal does not always yield better results.
- The body stores protein primarily in muscle, which serves as its only functional reserve. Protein cannot be derived from fat stores.
- Protein is meant for building and repairing tissues instead of being used as an expensive source of energy.
- Insulin plays a protective role by reducing muscle breakdown, helping preserve what protein is built.
- Protein quality, quantity and timing matter.
- The RDA for protein is 0.8 g/kg of body weight, which is essential to prevent deficiencies. It is for survival. However, to truly thrive, consume a minimum of 1–1.2 g/kg of body weight.
- Calories per gram of protein is a simple way to assess real protein value.
- Nutrition works best when nutrients work together rather than in isolation.

A Note from Me to You

If there is one key takeaway from this chapter, it is this: while protein is an important macronutrient, it is not magical or a superfood on its own. Every nutrient has its place in a balanced diet, provided it is consumed in the right amounts. Protein is not just about the numbers, grams, or labels; it is about how your body actually uses it. Consuming more protein does not automatically lead to better results. The emphasis on protein often arises because the typical Indian diet tends to be higher in carbohydrates and fats. Protein matters, but so do its timing, quality, and context. It is meant to build and repair, not to be burned as fuel. Nutrition works best when nutrients work together, rather than in isolation. Choose balance over extremes.

Habit 8

Protein at every meal

Incorporating a salad before meals improves fibre intake with little effort. Similarly, developing a protein habit does not require meticulously counting grams or changing your diet.

The key to this habit is simple: ensure each meal includes a clear source of protein.

Before you start eating, take a moment to ask yourself: What is the protein on this plate?

The source could be eggs, dairy, lentils, tofu, fish, meat, or a thoughtfully planned combination of foods. Dairy products, for this reason, often come in handy. If a meal consists only of *sabzi* and *roti*, adding half to one cup of curd alongside it can balance the plate.

Similarly, if you are eating sprouts, adding a tablespoon of soya granules or some *paneer* can improve the overall protein quality. Breakfast options like *poha* or *upma* are largely carbohydrate-based[12], so complementing them with a glass of milk or a bowl of curd can help complete the meal.

This does not mean you should overload your meals or eliminate other components. It simply means that protein should be included as a regular part of your diet rather than being seen as optional. When protein becomes a regular part of meals, muscle repair, satiety, and recovery begin to take care of themselves naturally.[13]

There is no need to complicate things or rush into excessive protein consumption. Do not overload every meal; one sensible serving of protein is enough to begin with. Give your body time to adjust.

Track Your Progress

Pause Again. On Purpose

Congratulations on completing eight chapters! If it seems like another pause is coming up too soon, that is intentional.

Nutrition does not change simply through acquiring information; it changes through repetition, awareness and small course corrections. Taking the time to review your progress at this point will help you identify patterns that may not have been clear before, especially after gaining a deeper understanding of protein and how it plays a role in daily meals.

Go back to the 'Track Your Progress' section from Chapter 3 once again. Record the same markers and compare them with:

- where you started, and
- your last check-in.

This is not about achieving faster results. It is about recognising how your body responds when fundamentals begin to settle in.

Each check-in shifts more responsibility from instructions on a page to your own observations. Over time, this is what builds confidence and food freedom.

So, track these again.

Daily measurements

- Water intake: ______ litres per day
- Sleep duration: ______ hours per day
- Sleep quality: Poor/Good/Excellent
- Energy levels throughout the day: Poor/Good/Excellent

Weekly assessments

- Sugar cravings: High/Moderate/None
- Hunger pangs/craving for snacks: Often/Moderate/Rarely
- Bowel movement: Regular/Constipation/Frequent indigestion
- Flatulence/gas/acidity/heartburn: Severe/Moderate/Rarely

Note: If you have not already, start tracking your girth measurements weekly. You may check your weight daily, not to react to fluctuations but to learn how your body responds to food, sleep, and routine over time.

9

Fats: Fats Do Not Make You Fat

The Misunderstood Case of Fat

For decades, like carbohydrates and proteins, dietary fat has been a subject of disputes and shifting narratives.

At first, fat was cast as the villain of the nutrition world. The logic seemed simple: since fat is calorie-dense, consuming fat must lead to weight gain. This belief shaped low-fat dietary guidelines, filled supermarket shelves with 'fat-free' products, and caused an entire generation to fear *ghee*, butter and oil.

The pendulum then swung to the opposite extreme, with fats being praised and, in some cases, labelled as superfoods.

> **Before understanding how fat works in the body, it helps to understand why it was misunderstood in the first place.**

The problem is that biology does not work in straight lines. Fat alone does not cause obesity; rather, chronic excess calorie intake does. Even then, obesity is multifactorial, influenced by refined carbohydrate intake, low physical activity, metabolic health, stress, and sleep.

Ironically, when fat was removed from foods, it was often replaced with sugar and starch to maintain taste. This resulted in poorer satiety, higher intake, and unstable blood sugar levels, which was hardly an improvement.

In today's world, we often feel compelled to make foods compete with one another, assigning them labels like 'good', 'bad', 'healthy' or 'superfood'. But food was never meant to compete; it is meant to fuel us, sustain us, and connect us to culture and routine.

True health is built through a combination of foods and consistent eating habits, rather than relying on a single standout ingredient.

From a Physiological Standpoint

Fat is not just a source of energy; it is also a crucial structural nutrient,[1] a signalling molecule, and a supporter of hormonal functions. Removing fat indiscriminately is like removing oil from an engine to prevent leaks; it does not solve the problem but instead damages the system.

Understanding this historical context is important because many people still harbour an unconscious fear of fats. Before learning about the benefits of fats, we need to unlearn the reasons we were taught to fear them.

What Dietary Fat Is

- **As a macronutrient:** Dietary fat is a macronutrient composed of fatty acids. While it is calorie (energy)-dense, providing 9 calories per gram (9 kcal/gm), reducing fat to 'just calories' overlooks its important functions.
- **For cell structure:** Fats are integral to cell membranes, which means every cell in your body, from muscles

to the brain, depends on fat for both structure and communication. Without adequate fat, cells can become rigid or fragile, much like a soap bubble without enough elasticity and strength.

- **As a fuel:** Fat also acts as a slow-burning fuel, meaning it digests gradually and provides sustained energy. This is why meals that contain some fat keep you feeling full longer than carb-only meals. Think of carbohydrates as kindling: they light fast and burn fast. In contrast, fat acts like a log that keeps the fire steady.

Fat is not just an energy source, it is a functional nutrient with structural and regulatory roles.

- **As a carrier:** Importantly, fats play an important role as carriers. Vitamins A, D, E and K are fat-soluble, meaning they are poorly absorbed without the presence of fat. Therefore, even the healthiest salad becomes nutritionally incomplete if it does not include any accompanying fat.

Understanding fat as a functional nutrient rather than just an energy source changes how we include it in meals.

Functions of Fat

Some roles of fat cannot be replaced by carbohydrates or proteins, regardless of calorie intake.

Fat plays roles that carbohydrates and proteins simply cannot fully replace. One of its most critical functions is hormone production. Many hormones, especially steroid hormones like oestrogen, testosterone, and cortisol, are synthesised from cholesterol and fatty acids. Following a chronically low-fat diet can lead to hormonal irregularities, poor recovery, or menstrual disturbances.

Fat is also essential for the nervous system. The brain is composed of nearly 60 per cent fat by dry weight. When fat intake is inadequate or imbalanced, people often report brain fog, mood changes, and poor focus. This occurs not because fat is magical, but because its structure matters.

Another major role of fat is satiety. Fat slows down gastric emptying,[2] meaning food remains in the stomach longer, sending fullness signals to the brain. As a result, meals that contain fat tend to feel more satisfying and emotionally complete.

Finally, fat provides insulation and protection. Body fat cushions organs and helps regulate temperature. It is not decorative storage; it is a functional reserve. Just like savings in a bank, body fat exists to support survival, not to be eliminated recklessly.

Types of Fats: Not All Fats Behave the Same

Classifying all fats into a single category is like calling all vehicles 'transport' without distinguishing between bicycles, cars, and trucks. While they all move you, the way they achieve this is important.

Fats differ in their structure, which determines how they function in the body.

Additionally, individuals respond differently to the same fat intake based on factors such as age, gender, and lifestyle. For instance, a physically active person, a sedentary person, a perimenopausal woman, and an endurance athlete will all respond differently to the same intake of fat. Metabolic health, gut health, and overall diet composition influence outcomes far more than fat alone.

Fats can be broadly divided into two categories:

- **Saturated fats:** These fats are more stable.
- **Unsaturated fats:** These fats are more flexible.

This structural difference affects digestion, oxidation, inflammation, and hormone signalling.

Unsaturated fats are further divided into two categories:

- Monounsaturated fats (MUFA)
- Polyunsaturated fats (PUFA)

Instead of asking 'Is fat good or bad?', a better question to consider is: Which fat should I consume, in what amounts, and in what context?

Not all fats behave the same; their structure determines their stability, function, and impact.

There is no single, fixed ratio of fat types to consume; the goal is optimal balance and variety, not equal proportions.

This means that no type of fat is inherently better than the other; none is a hero nor a villain. Your body requires a variety of fats in equal ratios to maintain harmony.

Striving for perfection can be unrealistic. Hence, it is best to focus on consuming a diverse range of fats rather than fixating on just one type. Consume all without biases.

By understanding different types of fats, we can use them more strategically rather than being influenced by emotions or past experiences. This perspective helps shift our focus from nostalgia or fear to functionality.

The Room Analogy (Part 1)

Building a room with different materials

Think of your body as a building, with every cell representing a room inside that building.

To function properly, each room needs four walls, not all of which are made of the same material, but are selected for a specific purpose.

For example:

- Brick walls make up most of the structure; they are strong, solid and dependable.
- Glass windows allow light in and facilitate communication with the outside world, but they are fragile and require careful placement.
- A wooden door enables controlled entry and exit; it is sturdy, flexible, and functional.

Together, these materials create one complete functional room. None of these is 'better' than the other; each serves a purpose. If you were to attempt to build the entire room using only one type of material, the result would likely be too rigid, too fragile, or simply impractical.

Dietary fats work in a similar way.

Saturated fats, MUFAs and PUFAs are not competing with each other. Instead, they act as different building materials within the same system. Their distinct structure determines how they behave, how stable they are and what role they play. Now, with this analogy, let us decode the three types of fats.

To gain a better understanding of fats, let us create a clearer picture.

Saturated Fats: The Brick Wall

Saturated fats are like brick walls; they are strong, stable, and provide structure.

These fats are primarily found in animal products such as butter, *ghee*, dairy fat, egg yolks, and meat. Coconut is a notable plant source of saturated fat. Structurally, these fats are solid at room temperature.

Think of fats as building materials: strength, flexibility, and communication all require different components.

In the body, saturated fats provide structural support to cell membranes, help cells maintain shape, and support the production of certain hormones. Due to their chemical structure, saturated fats are more resistant to heat and oxidation, which is why fats like *ghee*, butter, and coconut oil perform well during cooking.

Brick walls are not decorative; they are foundational.

But imagine building every wall, window, and door using only bricks. The room would be sturdy, yes, but dark, rigid, and poorly adaptable.

Similarly, saturated fats are necessary, but excess intake, especially without physical activity or a balanced diet, can reduce cellular flexibility. They work best when they form part of the structure, not the entire structure. So they are not inherently inflammatory, as once believed.

Stability gives structure, but too much rigidity reduces adaptability.

Context determines outcome:[3] For most healthy, active individuals, moderate saturated fat intake from whole foods is not a problem. The problem is rarely *ghee* alone; it is how much *ghee* is combined with excess sugar, refined flour, inactivity and stress.

Unsaturated Fats: Access Points

Unsaturated fats are liquid at room temperature and have a more flexible structure. They play a key role in metabolic regulation, cell signalling, and cardiovascular health.

These fats are generally seen as protective, but nuance still matters. Unsaturated fats are more likely to oxidise, especially when overheated or overused. Therefore, quality, storage and cooking method become important.

Unsaturated fats are further divided into MUFAs and PUFAs, each with different roles.

MUFAs: The Wooden Door

MUFAs are like a wooden door—strong, flexible, and functional.

They are found in foods like olive oil, mustard oil, avocados, peanuts, almonds, and certain seeds. These fats are often described as the 'middle ground': stable enough for moderate cooking and beneficial for metabolic health.

The wooden door is not meant to create a rigid barrier but to allow controlled entry and exit. Wood is durable yet adaptable. It does not shatter like glass or harden like brick.

But imagine a room filled with doors everywhere, with no sturdy walls or glass windows. The room will be dark, with many entry and exit points, so it would lack both safety and light.

Similarly, MUFAs[4] support metabolic flexibility, insulin sensitivity and healthy lipid transport. These fats help cells respond properly to signals rather than becoming too rigid or inflamed.

They are like the all-rounder in a sports team: they are reliable, adaptable and rarely problematic, but they cannot win a match without the support of the key players. Similarly, MUFAs cannot function without the stability of the saturated fats and fluidity of the PUFAs.

These fats sit in the middle: stable enough for use, flexible enough for function.

But in practical terms, diets rich in MUFAs are generally easier to sustain. They improve flavour, satisfaction, and nutrient absorption without causing excessive inflammation or instability. They serve as the functional connector; not flashy, but essential.

PUFAs: The Glass Windows

PUFAs are like glass windows. They allow communication with the outside world: light, signals, and information, but they are also the most delicate.

Dietary sources of PUFA include fatty fish, nuts, seeds, and selected plant oils.

Their structure enables a strong response, making them powerful regulators in inflammation, immunity, and cell signalling. However, this power has a dual effect.

The most biologically active fats are also the most sensitive.

Glass is extremely useful, but it needs careful handling. Poor-quality glass cracks easily; too much exposure makes it weaker.

Similarly, PUFAs[5] are essential, but they are also highly sensitive to oxidation, heat, and imbalance. Their function depends greatly on quality, quantity, and ratio, not just consumption. They are necessary, but maintaining balance is critical.

PUFAs are where things get a bit more complex, as omega fats come into play..

These include omega-3, omega-6, and omega-9 fats. Omega-3 and omega-6 are essential fatty acids that must be obtained from the diet, while omega-9 is non-essential because the body can synthesise it internally.

Now, to understand them, let us complete the first picture: the room analogy.

The Room Analogy (Part 2)

Within the glass windows

Within the window, there can be different types of glass—some bringing balance and clarity, others creating issues when overused or poorly placed.

For instance:

- **Frosted glass:** High-quality and well-treated, it allows in soft, balanced light. It keeps the room bright without glare and creates a calm and comfortable space.
- **Clear glass:** Transparent and functional, it lets in bright light, but depending on the strength of the sun, it can also allow in excessive heat and glare, making the room uncomfortable despite being well built.
- **Carved glass:** Elegant, decorative glass is useful but optional; it provides additional value, without being necessary for basic functionality.

Now, let us apply this analogy to omega fats.

Omega-3 Fats: The Frosted Glass

Omega-3 fats are like frosted glass that allows light in without overheating the room and helps maintain a sense of balance inside.

In the body, omega-3 fats support calm communication, flexibility, and repair. They do not produce noise; they reduce it. When omega-3 intake is adequate, the internal environment tends to feel more stable and resilient.

Omega-3 fats are 'anti-inflammatory' and structurally critical for the brain, eyes and joints. They improve cell membrane fluidity, which boosts communication between cells. They are linked to better recovery.

Sources include fatty fish, flaxseeds, chia seeds, and walnuts. Omega-3s are especially important for people with high stress, joint issues, autoimmune conditions or heavy training loads.

There is an important distinction to note. Omega-3 fats come in different forms, each serving a slightly different role in the body.

- **ALA (Alpha-linolenic acid):** ALA is a plant-based omega-3 found in foods like flaxseeds, chia seeds, and walnuts. ALA supports cardiovascular health and baseline anti-inflammatory balance, and importantly, serves as a precursor, meaning the body must convert it into the more active form, EPA and DHA, a process that is often inefficient.
- **EPA (Eicosapentaenoic acid):** EPA is an active omega-3 found mainly in fatty fish that helps actively regulate inflammation and supports recovery, joint health, and cardiovascular function.
- **DHA[6] (Docosahexaenoic acid):** DHA is a structural omega-3 fatty acid found in fatty fish and algae. DHA is essential for brain, eye, and nervous system health, playing a key role in cognition, vision, and overall cellular integrity.

For those who do not eat fish or fish oil, algae-based omega-3 supplements can help meet these needs.

Remember, they do not function like painkillers; they operate like maintenance crews—quietly and gradually.

Modern diets often lack sufficient omega-3s due to lower intake of fatty fish, increased reliance on processed foods, and a higher consumption of omega-6-rich vegetable oils.

Omega-6 Fats: The Clear Glass

Omega-6 fats are like clear glass windows. They let in bright light—quickly and efficiently. This light is necessary. Without it, the room would be dim, unresponsive, and unable to react when needed.

In the body, omega-6 fats play a critical role in normal inflammatory responses,[7] which are essential for wound healing, injury repair, immune defence, and recovery from physical stress. In this context, inflammation is not damage; it is the body's repair signal.

Problems arise only when the room has too many large, clear windows that all face harsh sunlight. Similarly, omega-6 becomes problematic not because it exists, but because modern diets supply it in excessive and concentrated amounts—mainly from refined vegetable oils used in processed and commercially prepared foods—while omega-3 intake remains low.

In a balanced system, omega-6 initiates inflammation when needed, and omega-3 helps resolve it afterwards. Trouble begins only when initiation overwhelms resolution.

Omega-9: The Carved Glass

Omega-9 fats are like interior glass features, which are useful additions but not essential to the basic design. The building can produce or manage these elements on its own when the overall structure and materials are sufficient.

That is why omega-9 is supportive but considered non-essential. The body can synthesise it internally, and deficiency is rare. Dietary sources of omega-9 fatty acids, which are readily available in a balanced diet, help support overall health.

With omega fats, balance matters more than absolute intake.

So omega-9 fats are not the main focus like omega-3 and omega-6.

Omega-9 fats can be produced by the body and are usually sufficient in balanced diets. They are beneficial but rarely result in deficiency.

Omega Fats: Where Most Diets Go Wrong

Just as yin and yang coexist for harmony, omega-3 and omega-6 fats work together in the body.

Omega-3 aids in resolving inflammation, while omega-6 promotes inflammatory responses required for healing and repair. Health depends on a balance between the two, not the elimination of either.

From a physiological perspective, a ratio closer to 1:1 is often viewed as an ideal reference point. However, modern diets[8] are heavily skewed towards omega-6 fats, while omega-3 intake has declined significantly.

The problem is rarely deficiency or excess alone; it is disproportion.

This imbalance does not lead to immediate illness, but over time, it creates a persistent low-grade inflammatory environment. This is similar to background noise that does not stop the music but makes everything harder to hear. The solution is not to eliminate omega-6, which is essential, but rather to improve the balance by increasing omega-3 intake.

Trans Fats: They Deserve Avoidance, Not Balance

If there is one thing that I would tell you to avoid as much as possible, it is trans fat, not out of fear but with awareness.

Among all dietary fats, trans fats are the only type that offer no physiological benefit; on the contrary, they harm the body more. While other fats can support health depending on their quality, quantity and context, trans fats are fundamentally different in how the body processes them.

What Are Trans Fats?

Trans fats are unsaturated fats that have been chemically altered through partial hydrogenation. This industrial process converts liquid vegetable oils into semi-solid fats, making them resemble *ghee* and butter—the saturated fats. They look similar but do not function the same way inside the body. They are structurally altered versions that behave differently in the body.

They are commercially used because they are inexpensive, improve mouthfeel, withstand repeated heating, and extend shelf life. This has made them common in bakery products, packaged snacks, *vanaspati*, margarine, fried foods and street foods made with reused oil.

The problem is that human metabolism is not adapted to process this industrial trans fat efficiently, so doing so carries a physiological cost.

How Do Industrial Trans Fats Harm?[9]

- Worsen lipid profiles by raising LDL (bad cholesterol) and lowering HDL (good cholesterol).
- Promote chronic inflammation, independent of quantity.
- Impair blood vessel function and endothelial health.
- Disrupt insulin signalling, contributing to metabolic dysfunction.
- Alter cell membrane fluidity, affecting normal cellular communication.

Trans fats do not need balancing; they need minimising.

Unlike omega-6 fats, which become problematic mainly when consumed in excess, trans fats are inherently disruptive.

Small amounts of naturally occurring trans fats are found in dairy and meat from ruminant animals, but these are structurally different, present in very low quantities, and are not linked to the same health risks as industrially produced trans fats.

So, the bottom line on trans fats is that they are not a matter of moderation or balance. They are about minimising them, not obsessing over them.

Cooking Oils: Choosing Based on Stability, Not Trends

An oil's health impact depends more on how it is used than where it comes from.

One of the biggest mistakes in modern nutrition is selecting cooking oils based on marketing, trends, or single nutrients, instead of their stability and intended use.

Not all oils are suitable for all temperatures. Heating unstable oils is like driving a Formula-1 race car on a rocky road; it is not designed for that.

High-heat cooking requires stability.

Raw use demands freshness.

Understanding this prevents oxidative damage and inflammation.

Oil is not 'healthy' or 'unhealthy' in isolation.

So instead of asking, 'Which oil is the healthiest?', ask: 'Which oil should I use under so-and-so cooking condition?'

Factors to Look at While Choosing the Right Fat/Oil

- **Degree of saturation:** More saturated means more heat stable; more unsaturated means more fragile.
- **Smoke point:** The temperature at which oil starts to break down, though smoke point alone is not enough, as oxidation can begin even before the oil smokes.
- **Fatty acid structure:** PUFAs oxidise fastest, and it is these oxidised fats that increase inflammation and cellular stress.

Purpose-based Oil/Fat Selection

- **High heat/frying/tadka:** *ghee*, coconut oil for flavour and high-heat cooking, and butter for flavour or finishing.
- **Daily cooking/curries/*sabzi*s:** mustard oil, groundnut oil and sesame seed oil are suitable for longer cooking.
- **Light cooking:** olive oil.
- **Salads/finishing:** extra virgin olive oil, flaxseed oil, walnut oil.

PUFA oils that need caution due to their high omega-6 content include sunflower oil, safflower oil, soybean oil and rice bran oil. These oils are less heat-stable and oxidise easily.[10] They are not exactly 'toxic' as they are often portrayed, but they should not be used as the primary daily cooking oils, especially for high-heat cooking.

Fat storage is hormonally regulated, not fat-driven.

Remember, no single oil can do everything well. Oils should be chosen the same way we choose footwear: running shoes for running, slippers for home and formal shoes for work.

When oils are chosen based on stability, context, and tradition, fat stops being confusing and starts becoming functional.

Fat and Metabolic Health

Eating fat does not automatically lead to fat gain. Excess calories do.

Fat storage is controlled by hormones. When insulin remains chronically elevated due to frequent refined carbohydrate intake and excess calories, fat storage increases regardless of dietary fat intake.

Fat in Special Populations

Women, athletes, and people with thyroid or autoimmune issues often suffer the most from overly restrictive fat intake. Hormonal balance, recovery, and nervous system health depend heavily on adequate fat.

How Much Fat Do You Actually Need?

While there is no perfect, fixed number, here is a reference based on the World Health Organization (WHO) guidelines[11] on dietary fat intake:

Total fat: Adults should limit their total fat intake to about 30 per cent of total daily energy.

Saturated fats: Keep intake below 10 per cent of total daily energy intake and reduce consumption.

Omega balance: Focus on restoring balance by increasing omega-3 intake rather than eliminating omega-6 entirely.

Trans fats: These should be kept as low as possible, ideally below 1 per cent of total daily energy intake, and efforts should be made to eliminate industrially produced trans fats.

Focus: Prioritise unsaturated fatty acids (MUFAs and PUFAs) from plant sources.

Caution: A practical point to consider is cumulative intake. In many Indian diets, saturated fat already comes from milk, curd, *paneer*, eggs, and other animal foods. When these are combined with the liberal use of *ghee* or butter in cooking, total saturated fat intake can easily exceed recommended levels unintentionally. So now you know that *ghee* is not a superfood as it is often portrayed.

Recommendations vary based on age, gender, fitness and health goals. Signs of too little fat include poor satiety, hormonal issues, dry skin and low energy. Signs of excess fat include calorie overload and digestive discomfort.

Guidelines provide boundaries, not personalised prescriptions.

Practical Takeaway

Rotate fat sources. Prioritise omega-3s. Respect cooking methods. Eat fat with intention, not fear. Aim for balance rather than precision.

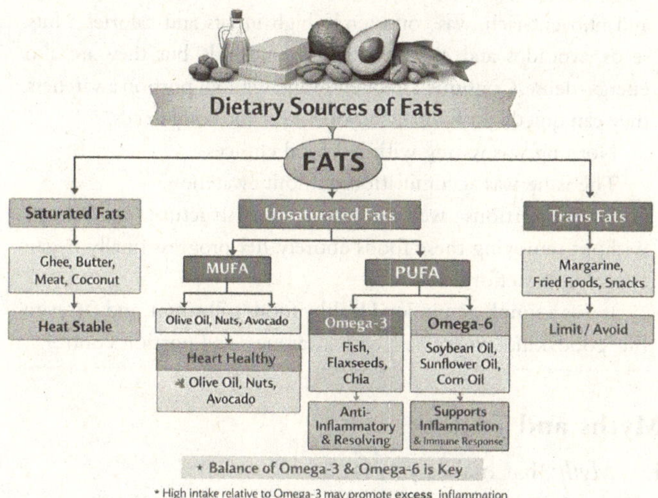

Figure 9.1: *Types of dietary fats and their common food sources*

Anecdote 11

Healthy choices, unintended accumulation

Even healthy choices can backfire when portion awareness is missing.

One of my clients, a forty-two-year-old woman, came to me genuinely confused.

'I eat only healthy food,' she said, 'but I am still gaining fat.'

When I reviewed her food log, nothing looked obviously unhealthy.

She ate one avocado almost every day, generous portions of guacamole, and added nuts and seeds liberally to her salads. When she stepped out, she avoided eating outside and instead ate nuts.

And she said that she used only *ghee* in her cooking.

When I asked her why, she replied, 'Because *ghee* is a superfood, it keeps the gut healthy and the joints also lubricated.'

None of these choices felt indulgent or imbalanced to her. In her mind, they were all 'healthy' foods.

But taken together, the pattern was clear. Her diet, though clean and nutrient-rich, was consistently high in fats and calories. Nuts, seeds, avocados and *ghee* are all valuable foods, but they are also energy-dense. Consumed frequently and without portion awareness, they can quietly push intake beyond what the body needs.

Nothing was wrong with her food choices.

The issue was accumulation without awareness.

Once portions were adjusted and structure introduced, without removing these foods entirely, her progress finally began to match her effort.

It was a simple reminder: Healthy foods still count, and fat, even the 'good' kind, works best with awareness and portion control.

Myths and Truths

1. *Myth:* 'Fat makes you fat.'

   Truth: Body fat gain is driven by overall calorie excess, not fat alone. Fat is calorie-dense, but when used appropriately, it can improve satiety and actually help regulate intake.

2. *Myth:* '*Ghee* is a superfood.'

   Truth: This is not true. *Ghee* is useful for cooking but does not provide a health benefit, especially in diets already high in saturated fat from full-fat dairy and other animal products. Labelling it a superfood can quietly encourage excess consumption.

3. *Myth:* 'All saturated fats are bad.'

   Truth: Saturated fats are not toxic. They are stable and useful for certain cooking methods. The issue is excess and stacking multiple saturated-fat sources, not moderate use of *ghee*, butter, or dairy.

4. *Myth:* 'More omega-3 automatically means better health.'

   Truth: Omega-3 is beneficial, but it works best when it balances omega-6 intake. Simply adding omega-3 without reducing excessive omega-6 does not fix inflammation.
5. *Myth:* 'Extra virgin oils are the best for cooking.'

   Truth: Extra virgin oils are nutritional oils, not cooking oils. Heating them destroys their antioxidants and can create oxidation products. They are best used cold or as finishing oils.
6. *Myth:* 'Low-fat diets are always healthier.'

   Truth: Very low-fat diets can reduce satiety, hormone production, skin health and energy levels, especially in active individuals and women. Fat is essential; the goal is an appropriate amount and quality, not elimination.
7. *Myth:* 'Homemade *makhan* can be used liberally because it has no chemicals.'

   Truth: Everything we eat is chemical in nature. Being homemade does not change its fat profile, and using it liberally, especially with full-fat dairy, can easily push saturated fat intake beyond healthy limits.
8. *Myth:* '*Ghee* lubricates the joints and is good for joint health.'

   Truth: Ghee does not reach the joints to lubricate them. Joints are lubricated internally by synovial fluid. While fat is important for overall health, adding extra *ghee* mainly increases calorie and saturated fat intake. Joint structure and repair depend more on adequate protein intake, along with movement and hydration, than on dietary fat.

9. *Myth:* 'Seed oils are bad for health.'

   Truth: Seed oils are flexible because their unsaturated structure supports cell communication and immune responses; problems arise from excess, imbalance, and overheating, not from their presence alone.

10. *Myth:* 'Bulletproof coffee (coffee with *ghee*/butter) is a healthy morning ritual.'

    Truth: Any appetite suppression from bulletproof coffee, if it happens at all, mainly comes from caffeine, which is a known appetite suppressant. Adding *ghee* only increases calories and saturated fat; it does not provide additional nutritional benefits.

    If someone thinks it boosts metabolism or gives an instant surge of energy, that too is a misconception. Fats digest slowly and are absorbed later in the digestive process, so *ghee* does not provide rapid energy. Any immediate 'kick' after bulletproof coffee comes from caffeine, not from the fat.

Most fat myths come from oversimplification, selective evidence, and fear-based messaging used to push products or ideologies.

To Reiterate

- Fat does not cause fat gain; chronic calorie excess does.
- Dietary fat is a functional nutrient, essential for hormones, brain health, satiety, and nutrient absorption.
- No single food or fat is a superfood; health comes from patterns, not ingredients.
- Different fats behave differently; structure determines function and stability.
- Saturated fats, MUFAs and PUFAs are all important; they work best in balance, not in isolation.
- Omega fats require a better balance of omega-3 and omega-6.
- Trans fats are the exception and should be minimised as much as possible.
- Cooking oils should be chosen for stability and use, not trends or labels.
- 'Healthy' fats are still calorie-dense; portion awareness matters.
- The goal is balance over precision, guided by individual needs and context.

A Note from Me to You

Fat has never been the problem. It is our relationship with it that has been the problem.

This chapter is not about eating more or less fat but about understanding it well enough to stop fearing or glorifying it. When fats are chosen consciously and used in moderation, they support health quietly and effectively. Food was never meant to cause anxiety or strict rules; it exists to promote health, energy and everyday living.

If this chapter helps you move away from fear, excess, or unquestioned beliefs and closer to informed, practical choices, then it has fulfilled its purpose.

Habit 9

Balance fat quantity and quality

Step 1: Audit Fat First

Before making any changes, identify where dietary fat is already coming from. Pay particular attention to sources of saturated fat. In Indian diets, these often include full-fat and toned milk, curd, *paneer*, butter, *ghee*, coconut, egg yolks, and animal products like meat and poultry. When multiple sources are combined, saturated fat intake can rise quickly, unintentionally.

If you decide to include *ghee* or butter, do so intentionally rather than adding them on top of a base already high in saturated fats.

Step 2: Choose Dairy for Protein and Calcium, Not Fat

Milk and dairy products are primarily consumed for their protein and calcium content, not as a source of fat. Checking food labels and selecting lower-fat options (such as 1–2 per cent fat, double-toned milk, or low-fat curd) helps limit unintended saturated fat intake while maintaining nutritional benefits.

Avoid going completely fat-free (0 per cent), since a small amount of fat helps with the absorption of fat-soluble vitamins.

This simple switch allows for small amounts of *ghee* or butter without significantly increasing total fat intake.

Step 3: Shift the Fat Quality, Not Just the Quantity

Once saturated fat intake is controlled, focus on improving fat quality. Increase intake of MUFAs (such as mustard oil, groundnut oil, and olive oil) and omega-3 fats through dietary sources. If fish is not part of the diet, consider omega-3 supplements (fish oil or algae oil) to meet EPA and DHA needs.

The goal is not to have a high-fat diet, but to achieve a better balance, so that total fat stays moderate while the fatty acid profile improves.

A balanced Indian diet is not achieved by removing fat entirely, but by limiting excess saturated fat, improving fat quality, and keeping total fat moderate and intentional.

With this chapter, we complete the basics of good nutrition. From here, we focus on arranging your plate for better balance and nourishment.

Track Your Progress

A Brief Check-In

You have now completed nine chapters, covering carbohydrates, proteins and fats. Before moving ahead, take a moment to notice how these changes are showing up in your daily life.

This is, once again, a simple review, not an evaluation. Revisiting the same markers helps you stay on track. There is nothing quite as motivating as noticing subtle shifts in energy, appetite or cravings. And even if there are no visible changes, this check-in helps set clear expectations.

Go to the 'Track Your Progress' section in Chapter 3 and record the same details again.

Compare them with:

- where you began, and
- your previous check-ins.

The goal here is to observe trends. These observations will make the upcoming chapters on structuring your plate and managing portions much easier to implement.

Remember Peter Drucker's statement?

'What gets measured gets managed!'

Daily measurements

- Water intake: ______ litres per day
- Sleep duration: ______ hours per day
- Sleep quality: Poor/Good/Excellent
- Energy levels throughout the day: Poor/Good/Excellent

Weekly assessments

- Sugar cravings: High/Moderate/None
- Hunger pangs/craving for snacks: Often/Moderate/Rarely
- Bowel movement: Regular/Constipation/Frequent indigestion
- Flatulence/gas/acidity/heartburn: Severe/Moderate/Rarely

Taking Your Measurements

Along with the check-in, this is also a good time to record your physical measurements again.

Use the same method you followed in Chapter 3 so that comparisons stay meaningful. Take these measurements first thing in the morning after freshening up, and ideally in light clothing.

Today's Date: ____________ **Weight:** ____________

Please take the following measurements using a measuring tape (in inches or cm):

Body Part	Measurement	Body Part	Measurement
Neck	________	Shoulder	________
Chest	________	Biceps	________
Waist (narrowest part)	________	Waist (belly button)	________
Waist (2 inches below belly button)	________	Hips	________
Thigh	________	Calf	________

Table 9.1: *Recommended body measurement points for tracking changes in body composition over time*

10

Structuring Your Plate

YOU NOW UNDERSTAND CARBOHYDRATES, proteins and fats not as isolated villains or heroes, but as nutrients that play specific roles in the body. The next step is to learn how to combine them together in a way that supports your health, fitness goals and lifestyle. This is where structuring your plate comes into play.

Structuring your plate is not about eating less.

It is not about cutting foods out.

And it is certainly not about creating rigid food rules.

It is about composition, not restriction.

This chapter connects nutrition theory to everyday eating. It aims to simplify decisions, not add extra work to your routine or overwhelm you when you are busy or travelling. The goal is to clear up confusion and help you eat mindfully.

There is no need to focus on portion control or calorie counting here. Before changing portion sizes, it is important to first understand what a well-structured meal looks like.

Most people struggle with food, not because they eat too much but because their meals lack structure. A plate without adequate protein often leaves you hungry soon after. Meals high in refined carbohydrates without enough fibre or fat can cause energy crashes. Meals that lack volume or satisfaction tend to trigger grazing and cravings later. None of this requires more willpower; it requires better structure.

The goal is not perfection but consistency with ease.

Instead of asking, 'How much should I eat?' at every meal, consider asking, 'Does this plate have what I need?'

Once the structure is in place, feedback becomes easier to interpret.

Your progress tracking is simply your body responding. If cravings remain unchanged, hunger peaks in the evening, or energy dips happen in the afternoon, it may be a sign that your meals need to be better structured.

Hydration, fibre-rich foods and regular protein intake all help. But if you are still struggling, take a moment to review whether you have been applying these habits consistently. These habits are designed to build gradually, allowing results to emerge over time.

Do not get discouraged if changes feel slow. Pause, observe, and re-assess.

By the end of the chapter on fats, you should already have a clear understanding of how your three main meals—breakfast, lunch and dinner—can be structured. If you include one to three snacks, those are best built around protein and fibre.

This structure creates predictability for both you and your body. The human body thrives on routines: regular fuel, balanced inputs, and meals that promote both physical satiety and mental satisfaction. When meals are consistently balanced, the body does not need to compensate later through cravings, fatigue or loss of control around food.

This is why plate structure precedes portion control. Without structure, portion control feels forced. With structure, it becomes intuitive.

Structure does not mean a strict rulebook.

A structured plate is meant to be a default setting, not a rigid template you must follow every time you eat.

It represents how you eat most of the time, not all the time.

There will be lighter meals.

There will be indulgent meals.

There will be meals eaten socially, emotionally, or simply for pleasure.

Structure does not remove flexibility; it creates room for it.

When your daily meals are generally balanced, occasional unstructured meals no longer feel disruptive.

Structure Supports Both Physical and Mental Satiety

You might have heard the familiar line, '*Pet bhar gaya, par mann nahi bhara.*'

It is often said as a compliment to the person who cooked the meal, but it also captures something deeper about how we eat. I like to say, '*Pet bhi bharo, aur mann bhi.*' In other words, eat to satisfy all your senses.

Our senses are closely connected to the brain, and the brain prepares the body for food even before the first bite by releasing digestive enzymes and hormones.

- **Nose:** Aroma can trigger hunger instantly. Ever walked into a home and recognised the smell of your favourite food? Your appetite responds even before you see the plate.

- **Eyes:** Visual cues matter. A plate that looks sparse can signal insufficiency, while a full-looking portion suggests fullness even before eating begins.
- **Ears:** The sounds of sizzling, crunching, or crackling food enhance the eating experience and indicate freshness and texture.
- **Skin:** Touch also matters—feeling warmth, cold, softness or a crunch sends sensory feedback to the brain.
- **Tongue:** Finally, taste completes the experience. When food tastes good, it elicits pleasure and satisfaction, influenced by both the food itself and your emotional state.

All five senses contribute to your satisfaction after a meal.

Eating slowly allows these signals to register. Chewing properly gives saliva, rich in digestive enzymes, time to mix with food, supporting digestion even before the food reaches the stomach.

A well-structured plate addresses both of these essential aspects of eating:

- **Physical satiety:** This comes from protein, fibre, adequate volume, and sufficient energy. These elements promote fullness, slow digestion, and help stabilise blood sugar.
- **Mental satisfaction:** This comes from taste, texture, familiarity, and enjoyment. Meals that ignore this often lead to cravings later, even if they are nutritionally 'perfect'.

Structuring your plate is about honouring both.

Nutrition works best when meals are both nourishing and enjoyable. When satisfaction is missing, the body keeps craving food, not out of greed but because something feels unfinished. When nutrition is neglected, fatigue follows, not because you ate less but because your body lacks structure.

Now, let us structure the plate.

Structuring your plate does not require new foods, special products, or complicated rules. It simply involves looking at what you already eat and bringing a little order to it.

Think of your plate as a framework, not a strict formula. It is meant to guide you, not control you. A well-structured plate answers four simple questions:

- Is there a clear source of protein?
- Is there a source of energy? Think grains or other carbohydrates.
- Is there enough volume and fibre? Think of vegetables or fruits.
- Is there enough variety to support digestion and enjoyment?

Fats are usually already present through cooking, tempering, spreads, or dressings, and do not always need separate attention at every meal.

You do not need all components in perfect proportion every time. If most meals include at least three of these elements, the plate is well-balanced enough.

This approach applies to home-cooked meals, dining out, travel and social occasions. The foods may change, but the structure remains the same. For now, avoid focusing on portions, calories or limits. This chapter is about completeness, not quantity. We will address how much and how often in the next section.

Before you start eating, take a moment to look over your plate and ask yourself, 'Is there anything missing here?'

If something is missing and easy to add, do so. If not, eat and think about balancing it later in the day. What you do most of the time is much more important than doing everything perfectly for a short time and risking burnout. Consistency matters more than perfection.

Time To Bring the Habits Together

So far, each chapter has introduced a small, focused habit. On its own, each habit may have seemed simple, perhaps even repetitive. That, as you know by now, was intentional.

You were never meant to practise these habits in isolation forever.

As you begin structuring your plate, these habits naturally come together. What once required conscious effort now feels automatic. You may already notice how these habits quietly answer the questions of a structured plate we just discussed:

- Starting meals with vegetables improves fibre intake and supports digestion.
- Including a visible protein source helps boost satiety and steady energy levels.
- Being aware of fat sources prevents unintentional stacking, without restrictions.

When these habits work together, the plate begins to organise itself.

In most Indian diets, grains have traditionally been abundant. The focus, therefore, was never on adding more grains but on improving balance by bringing vegetables and protein to the plate. Without this shift, reducing excess grains would not be practical or sustainable.

At this stage, you are no longer asking, 'Am I doing this right?'

You are simply preparing meals with mindfulness.

This is how structure forms, not through new rules but through habits working in sync. If these habits still do not feel automatic yet, keep practising them. A quick look at your plate will now be enough to tell you whether it is balanced or needs a small adjustment.

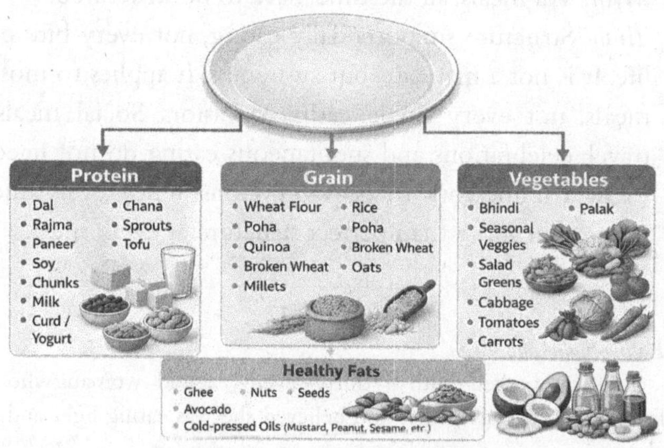

Figure 10.1: *Components of a balance*

Myths and Truths

1. *Myth:* 'A structured plate is rigid and boring.'

   Truth: Structure does not limit food choices; it supports flexibility and removes guesswork and guilt. The foods can change daily; the framework stays the same.

2. *Myth:* 'A structured plate means eating the same foods every day.'
   Truth: Structure refers to how a meal is put together, not which foods are chosen. Variety can be part of the same structure. Different cuisines, seasonal foods, home-cooked meals, restaurant meals, and social eating can all fit the same plate framework. The foods may change; the structure remains.
3. *Myth:* 'Bland, tasteless food means healthy food.'
   Truth: Health and flavour are not opposites. Enjoyment, aroma, texture, and familiarity all add to satisfaction. Meals that ignore taste often lead to cravings later, even if they are nutritionally balanced.
4. *Myth:* 'All meals, all the time, have to be structured.'
   Truth: Structure supports daily eating, not every bite of life. It is not a mandate, but awareness. It applies to most meals, not every single eating occasion. Social meals, travel, celebrations and spontaneous eating do not need to fit a framework to be valid. Consistency over time matters far more than perfect structure at every meal.

Anecdote 12

Eating 'light' and 'clean'

I once worked with a thirty-seven-year-old woman who followed a vegetarian diet and believed she was eating light and clean.

Her breakfast usually consisted of *poha*, *upma*, or *roti* with *sabzi*. Dinner was almost always *roti* and *sabzi*. She avoided *dal* at night because she felt protein was 'heavy' and might affect digestion. On some days, she chose vegetable *pulao* for dinner, thinking it would be lighter and easier on the body.

Lunch was the only meal where she included *dal*, yoghurt, and a more complete combination.

Between meals, she snacked on fruits, believing they were the healthiest option. She also drank four to five cups of tea daily, each with milk and about two teaspoons of sugar, and had soaked nuts in the morning.

On paper, everything looked reasonable. There were no 'junk' foods, no overeating, no desserts, and no obvious excess. Yet she often felt hungry, especially in the evenings, and relied on frequent snacking and multiple cups of tea to get through the day, without realising how much sugar was adding up through beverages.

Upon closer inspection, the issue was not food quality but meal structure. Two of the three main meals lacked a clear protein source. Most of her energy came from carbohydrates, and protein was present in only one meal. The frequent fruit and tea were not improving her nutrition; they were merely compensating for incomplete meals.

We simply began bringing structure to her plates. As meals became more balanced, her urge to snack constantly decreased, and the multiple cups of tea naturally dropped.

The hunger did not settle because she ate less. It settled because her meals finally contained what they needed.

To Reiterate

- Structuring your plate is about composition, not restriction.
- A well-structured plate focuses on what is present, not what needs to be removed.
- Physical satiety and mental satisfaction are both essential for sustainable eating.
- Meals that lack structure are often the reason for cravings and low energy.
- A simple plate framework applies to home-cooked meals, eating out and travel.
- You do not need perfect proportions; most meals require only three of the four elements.
- Habits developed earlier naturally come together when you structure your plate.
- When the structure is consistent, portion control becomes intuitive rather than forced.

A Note from Me to You

If there is one thing I want you to take from this chapter, it is this: structure creates ease. You do not need strict rules or perfect meals to eat well. You need a plate that supports your body and satisfies your mind, most of the time. This chapter is not about control; it is about organisation. When meals are structured with awareness, energy feels steadier, cravings decrease, and hunger cues become clearer. Do not chase perfect plates. Build repeatable ones. Structure first, then add flexibility.

Habit 10

The plate pause

Before you begin eating, take a moment to pause and scan your plate.

Ask yourself just one question:

'What is missing here?'

Not what to remove.

Not how much to eat.

Just what is missing?

If something is easy to add, add it.

If not, eat and move on.

11

Portions and Goals: Putting the Pieces Together

WITH THIS CHAPTER, YOU come to the end of the basics of good nutrition.

So far, you have covered many concepts: physiology, nutrition science, food choices, and behaviour, mostly as separate topics. Each of these matters on its own, but nutrition does not work in isolation. Real progress happens when these pieces come together to create a bigger picture.

This chapter discusses integration.

It is where understanding turns into action and knowledge starts to produce results. When parts align with goals and choices are guided by awareness rather than strict rules, nutrition becomes practical, adaptable and sustainable.

Before discussing numbers, portions, or targets, we must return to the foundation on which they are built.

That foundation lies in awareness.

Awareness

Before we explore food portions further, I want to re-emphasise something I have been repeating throughout this book: Do not label food.

Food is not good or bad; it is just food.

Avoid labelling food 'good' or 'bad'. It is simply food.

Food has gradually become a moral issue. At some point, we stopped viewing it as nourishment and started assigning it labels—good, bad, clean, dirty, cheat, toxic, or even cruel. These labels may sound harmless, but they quietly shape how we eat, think, and feel about ourselves and others.

Food itself has not changed.

Our perception of it has changed.

What influences how food affects your health is not a single ingredient or meal, but the context, quantity, frequency, balance, beliefs, and your relationship with it.

Awareness helps you see food clearly: without fear, guilt, or extremes. Without awareness, portion control can feel restrictive, goals can feel stressful, and maintaining consistency becomes harder.

Context and consistency matter more than labels.

That is why this chapter begins here.

The Role of Thoughts and Messaging

Your thoughts and words about food can affect how your body responds to it.

This does not mean that thoughts change the calorie content of food. Calories remain the same. However, thoughts, emotions, and expectations can influence how the body processes and experiences a meal.

When food is constantly labelled as 'bad', 'unhealthy', or 'forbidden', it can cause stress and anxiety around eating. For some people, this increased stress may affect digestion, appetite control, gut motility and overall comfort after meals.

You may notice outcomes such as the following:

- Digestive discomfort
- Feeling heavy or sluggish
- Lower energy after eating
- Reduced enjoyment and satisfaction

This is not the food hurting you. It is your body reacting to a stressful eating environment, where the nervous system switches into a more protective, energy-saving mode.

When food is approached with neutrality and awareness, the body may respond differently. A calmer nervous system supports better digestion, clearer satiety signals, and a more stable energy response after meals.

Again, this does not change the number of calories or macronutrients.

What may change is:

- How comfortable you feel after eating.
- How satisfied you are.
- How your appetite behaves later in the day.

Over time, this can influence eating habits and consistency.

Awareness, therefore, is not passive.

It becomes meaningful once you begin noticing how your body responds.

Skill 1: Using Hunger Timing as Feedback

Once you remove fear and labels from food and learn to structure your plate better, the next step is to understand how your body responds to what you eat.

This is about understanding the language of the body.

The body reacts to every thought and action.

Now, let us put that into practice.

Notice how long a meal keeps you full before real hunger comes back.

A word of caution: Dehydration can sometimes feel like hunger and lead to cravings. Keep this in mind while observing.

This exercise is not about judging your food choices.

It is about recognising patterns to better understand your meals.

What Hunger Timing Can Tell You

- Sustains for a few hours

  Meals that include sufficient protein, moderate fat, fibre and volume tend to keep most people feeling full for a few hours.
- Hunger or cravings return quickly

  Meals high in carbohydrates, especially refined carbs, and low in protein and fat often cause hunger and cravings to return sooner.
- Energy crash

  Meals high in fat and carbohydrates but low in protein may feel heavy, decrease activity, and cause an energy dip.
- Heavy and full for too long

  This often occurs when vegetables are limited, and the meal consists of grains or protein with higher fat content. Eating too quickly can also be a factor.

If you notice that a meal makes you hungry again quickly or leaves you so full that you avoid food for hours, it usually signals that something was out of balance.

Using This Feedback

This hunger timing feedback can further help you to understand your plate better, and adjustments can be made accordingly in subsequent meals. For example:

- Adding more protein
- Adding fibre or volume with a salad
- Adjusting carbohydrates or fats

At this stage, do not ask: 'How much should I eat?' Instead, ask: 'How long did this meal actually sustain me?'

This approach teaches the following:

- Internal regulation
- Respect for hunger and fullness
- Adaptability across different days and schedules
- A natural transition into flexible eating

As a rough guide:

- Three to four hours of satiety usually indicates a well-balanced meal
- Five to six hours or more may suggest higher fat content
- Frequent hunger or constant snacking, including multiple teas or coffees with or without sugar and milk, may indicate meals higher in carbohydrates and lower in protein

This is not a rule; it is an observational skill that improves with practice, like any other skill.

Before moving to the next step, practise this for a few days. Focus on aligning with your body's cues rather than following only external instructions.

Skill 2: Using Structure When Awareness Is Difficult

Many people are too busy or mentally preoccupied to fully develop skill 1 initially. Some might even find it unsettling.

For those situations, here is skill 2, which ideally works best when used with skill 1.

I will provide you with a broad, context-based framework for macronutrient portions. These portions might vary depending on the following:

- Training versus rest days
- Age, gender and hormonal status
- Appetite, stress and sleep
- Lifestyle, culture and professional demands

A fixed ratio cannot capture all of this.

Most balanced diets naturally fall within a reasonable range of carbohydrates, proteins, and fats when meals are structured well. For most health goals, aiming for exact ratios is unnecessary.

The Numbers That Matter

Total Daily Calorie Intake

Your body responds first and foremost to total energy intake.

Whether your goal is to lose weight, gain muscle, or maintain weight, the number of calories you consume over time matters the most.

You can eat the healthiest foods available, but:

- If you consistently overeat, weight gain will occur.
- If you undereat, weight loss will occur.

- Chronic overeating and chronic undereating can both lead to fatigue, poor recovery, hormonal disruption and metabolic stress, though through different physiological pathways.

Calories are not the enemy. They are simply a measure of energy; think of them as a budget within which food choices are made.

No single day decides your outcome; your average intake over days and weeks does.

Tracking body weight and measurements weekly can help you adjust calories and macros appropriately.

Macronutrient Ratio

Calories tell you how much to eat.

Macronutrients determine how those calories are used.

Each macronutrient plays a distinct role:

- **Protein:** Muscle repair, recovery, immunity, satiety
- **Carbohydrates:** Training fuel, daily activity, brain function, hormonal balance
- **Fats:** Hormone production, nutrient absorption, joint and cellular health

Removing or excessively cutting any one of these creates an imbalance elsewhere.

A Practical Starting Framework

For most people, a sustainable macro range looks like:

- Carbohydrates: 45–55 per cent
- Protein: 20–30 per cent
- Fats: 20–30 per cent

This is not a rule; it is a starting point.

Why this works:

- Enough carbohydrates for energy and recovery
- Adequate protein to preserve or build muscle
- Sufficient fats for hormonal and long-term health

Once this foundation is in place, fine-tuning becomes much easier.

Connecting Numbers to the Balanced Plate

These numbers mostly align naturally with the half vegetables, one-fourth protein, one-fourth grains plate model for most people:

- Vegetables provide fibre, volume, and micronutrients
- Protein anchors meals and supports recovery
- Grains and starchy carbs provide energy
- Fats, though smaller in volume, are nutrient-dense and essential

When meals are consistently built this way, macro balance often takes care of itself.

Adjusting for Real Life

These ratios are not fixed:

- Higher training volumes may require more carbohydrates.
- Sedentary days may feel better with slightly lower carbs and higher protein.
- During fat loss phases, protein often shifts higher to control hunger.
- During stress or high-activity phases, carbohydrates may need to increase.

Vegetables
Broccoli, Salad,
Carrots, Peppers
Cooked Veggies
Protein
Chicken, Salmon,
Tofu, Eggs, Milk,
Dal, Lentils
Healthy Fats
Whole Grains
Brown Rice, Roti
& Bread, Millets, Rice

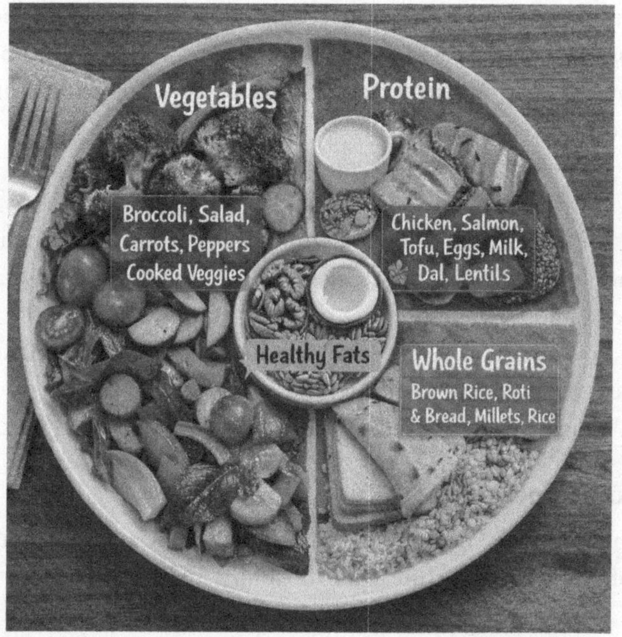

Figure 11.1: *Portion guide for a balanced plate*

Daily movement varies. Energy demands fluctuate. Flexibility matters.

The principle remains the same: meet your calorie needs first, then distribute macros intelligently. Do not reverse this order.

The Bigger Picture

Nutrition is not about perfect ratios or rigid rules. It is about:

- Meeting energy needs
- Fuelling performance
- Supporting recovery
- Maintaining long-term health

Numbers are tools, not commandments. When used correctly, they provide clarity, not control. They should be compared, cross-checked and adjusted to align with goals and feedback.

Now, awareness gives you clarity.

But clarity alone is not enough.

If eating becomes only about observation, measurement, and correction, it can still feel rigid and joyless. And what feels rigid rarely lasts.

For nutrition to be sustainable, it must leave room for pleasure, preference, culture, and life itself.

This is where soulfulness comes in.

Soulfulness

Soulfulness is not about ignoring awareness; it is about softening the structure with flexibility.

It recognises that food is not only fuel; it is also taste, memory, culture, celebration and connection. A plan that leaves no room for enjoyment eventually collapses, no matter how well-designed it is.

This balance is best explained through the 80:20 rule.

The 80:20 Rule

The 80:20 rule suggests the following:

- 80 per cent of the time, you focus on nourishing, well-balanced meals that support your health and goals.
- 20 per cent of the time, you allow space for foods that may be less nutrient-dense but are emotionally satisfying: foods that feel soulful.

This 20 per cent is not a 'cheat'.

It is intentional flexibility.

When flexibility is built in, deprivation reduces.

Planned enjoyment reduces rebellion.

When deprivation reduces, bingeing becomes less likely.

And when extremes disappear, consistency becomes easier.

This Is Not Set in Stone

The 80:20 framework is only a guideline, not a rulebook.

The ratio is not set in stone. Depending on your goals and life stage, it could be something like this:

- 90:10 during focused performance phases
- 80:20 for most people most of the time
- 70:30 during travel, festivals or high-stress periods

The principle behind it matters far more than the exact number.

The goal is to do better most of the time, without overwhelming yourself.

Common Diet Mistakes

Here are some of the most common mistakes I repeatedly see people make, often without realising that these habits hinder their progress.

Mistake 1: All or Nothing

Weekdays: All control.

Weekends: No control.

This is one of the most common patterns.

People eat 'perfectly' from Monday to Friday and then overindulge or overeat on weekends, holidays or travel days, believing they can reset everything again on Monday.

But your body does not follow a weekday–weekend schedule.

It follows biological rhythms: day and night cycles, seasons, recovery and consistency.

Your body does not reset:

- Every Monday
- After a holiday
- After travel
- After 'being good' all day and giving up at night

Your body responds to patterns, not to extremes.

It only understands what it receives consistently.

When weekdays are restrictive and weekends are excessive, the weekly average often cancels itself out. This leads to frustration, plateaus, and the false belief that nothing is working.

Consistency beats intensity every time.

One Meal Does Not Define Your Health

No single meal can:

- Ruin your progress
- Cause fat gain
- Destroy your metabolism
- Undo months of work

Just as one healthy meal does not make you fit, one indulgent meal does not make you unhealthy.

What matters over time is:

- Your average calorie intake

- Your protein adequacy
- Your fibre intake
- The quality of fats you consume
- How well you recover, sleep, and manage stress

Zoom out. Always look at the bigger picture.

Mistake 2: 'Earning' Your Food

Food is not a reward for burning calories.

Exercise is not punishment for eating.

When people feel they must 'earn' their meals:

- Movement becomes transactional
- Food becomes an obligation
- Hunger turns into cravings and deprivation
- Eating becomes emotionally loaded

You eat because your body needs fuel, nutrients, and energy to function, not as a reward for completing a workout or reaching a step count.

This change in mindset alone can significantly improve your long-term commitment and your relationship with food.

Mistake 3: Over-Doing One Macronutrient

This is a mistake I see often.

Non-vegetarians tend to overconsume protein because animal foods provide higher protein per gram. While protein intake remains high, fibre intake drops. When one macronutrient dominates the plate, another important component usually gets pushed out.

Vegetarians, on the other hand, often reach fibre goals more easily but struggle to get enough protein.

So, do not take sides—eat without bias.

No single food group is inherently superior.

And no single food is solely responsible for success or failure.

Balance matters more than allegiance.

Mistake 4: Making the Diet Exclusive

The most sustainable diets are inclusive rather than exclusive or restrictive.

When you allow a wider range of foods:

- Nutrient adequacy improves
- Cravings reduce
- Social life becomes easier
- Anxiety around food decreases

Avoid excluding entire food groups based on trends or hype without medical or ethical justifications, as it often adds unnecessary complexity. It can also increase the risk of nutrient deficiencies and overeating to compensate.

Eat everything that is real and edible, in appropriate portions, with awareness.

Balance does not mean eating everything all the time.

It means nothing is completely off-limits.

Mistake 5: Ignoring Hydration While Increasing Protein and Fibre

Increasing protein or fibre without increasing water intake is a very common oversight. Consuming more protein leads to more metabolic waste, increasing the body's water requirement.

Similarly, increasing fibre without sufficient water can impair gut motility.

Fibre works best in the presence of water. More fibre with less water can lead to constipation and poor gut health.

The same applies to supplements like creatine monohydrate; water intake should increase alongside them.

Adequate protein and creatine do not harm the kidneys. Inadequate hydration, however, certainly can.

Mistake 6: Over-Snacking on 'Healthy' Foods

Many people depend heavily on nuts for snacking.

Replacing biscuits, *mathri*s or *namkeen*s with nuts is definitely a better choice, but over-reliance creates a new problem.

Nuts are:

- Small in volume
- High in calories
- Easy to overeat

They need to be counted and tracked, just like any other calorie-dense food.

The same applies to foods like avocados and coconut. While nutritious, they can quickly increase total calorie intake if eaten without awareness.

'Healthy' foods can still derail progress when portions are ignored.

Mistake 7: Extreme Calorie Deficits and the Yo-Yo Cycle

Another common mistake I often see is creating an extreme calorie deficit in the hope of faster results.

When the deficit becomes too severe:

- Hunger and food obsession increase
- Energy levels drop

- The risk of muscle loss rises
- Training performance declines
- Recovery suffers
- The approach eventually becomes unsustainable

As a result, most people cannot sustain this for long. When the restriction breaks, eating often swings in the opposite direction: overeating, loss of structure, or 'giving up' altogether.

This commonly leads to the following:

- Rapid weight regain
- Regaining more weight than was lost
- Frustration and loss of trust in the process
- Repeated dieting attempts

This is the classic yo-yo effect.

The problem is not the deficit itself. The issue is trying to force too much, too soon, beyond what the body can realistically handle.

Weight loss that cannot be maintained is not success; it is a temporary change.

The goal is to lose weight in a way you can sustain long enough for it to stay off.

Sustainable progress comes from moderate, manageable calorie deficits that allow habits to develop and the body to adapt.

Extreme restriction disregards awareness, removes soulfulness and ultimately damages sustainability.

Gentle Reminder

Alcohol: A Commonly Overlooked Variable

Alcohol is not food and does not provide nourishment. Regardless of the type—wine, beer or spirits—alcohol remains alcohol, and no form of alcohol is considered good for health.

Alcohol is not calorie-free. In fact, 1 gram of alcohol provides approximately 7 calories. These calories add to your total energy intake but provide no nutrition. What is often overlooked is not only the alcohol itself, but also what tends to accompany it—mixers, snacks and unplanned eating that may not be consciously counted.

This section is not about restriction or judgement but awareness. When progress stalls despite consistent effort, alcohol and its add-ons are often the missing variable.

This applies not only to alcohol but also to many overlooked habits discussed in this section.

Most diet struggles are not due to a lack of discipline.

They arise from misunderstood habits, extremes, and unconscious patterns.

Fixing these common mistakes does not require perfection; it requires awareness, balance, and consistency. And those are skills you can learn.

Supplements and Common Deficiencies: A Reality Check

Supplements are meant to supplement, not replace, food, habits, or consistency. They can play a supportive role when deficiencies exist or needs increase, especially for those who monitor weight, train regularly or play sports.

You do not need all supplements, but you also do not need to avoid them when there is a genuine need. Supplementation should always be guided by blood markers, not guesswork.

Vitamin D deficiency is common because of limited sun exposure and can affect bone health, immunity and recovery.

Vitamin B12 may be low in vegetarians or those with limited intake of animal food, and it can affect energy and nerve health.

Iron deficiency is common among women, leading to fatigue and reduced exercise tolerance.

Beyond these, calcium, magnesium and omega-3 fats can be beneficial depending on diet, training load, stress and recovery, and should be individualised.

The goal is not to take more supplements, but to identify gaps and address them intentionally.

Guilt-Free Eating Is Not Careless Eating

Eating without guilt does not mean eating without structure.

It means:

- You enjoy your meals without shame.
- You return to routine without punishment.
- You make choices based on information, not fear.
- You trust yourself to self-correct.

You stop 'earning' meals.

You stop punishing yourself for enjoyment.

You stop swinging between control and loss of control.

Instead, you build trust with food and with yourself.

Structure and flexibility can coexist. In fact, they are essential for long-term success.

Awareness without soulfulness becomes rigid.

Soulfulness without awareness becomes chaotic.

When the two work together, nutrition becomes liveable.

The Big Goal

Sustainability

Awareness + Soulfulness = Sustainability

Sustainability is not something you can force.

It is the result of alignment.

A diet that seems 'perfect' on paper but fails in real life is not a good diet.

The best diet is one you can stick to indefinitely. Most diets do not fail because people lack discipline but because life eventually intervenes. That is when most people get derailed, for instance:

- During busy weeks
- During celebrations
- During stress
- During normal, boring days
- Once a weight target is achieved

When the diet ends, accountability often disappears, whether it was to a plan, a coach or a rulebook. What usually follows is uncontrolled eating, loss of structure, and the start of yet another yo-yo dieting cycle.

But genuine health is built on sustainability, not on quick bursts of control.

Achieving Sustainability

Sustainability is achieved when:

- You treat your body with compassion.
- You introduce smaller, manageable changes.
- You build habits one at a time.
- You allow the body time to adapt.

- You stop punishing yourself with extreme workouts or rewarding yourself with excess.

Food was never meant to create fear, guilt or moral superiority.

It was meant to nourish, satisfy, connect and sustain you.

Reflect, adjust, continue. Do not restrict.

Drop the labels.

Drop the extremes.

Drop the all-or-nothing mindset.

Do better most of the time.

Stay flexible when life demands it.

And remember, health works best when it includes balance, not obsession.

Food is not good or bad.

It's just food.

Anecdote 13

Speed vs sustainability

About a decade ago, I coached a woman for fat loss. Over two to three years of consistent personal training, nutrition coaching, and gradual habit changes, she lost around 22–25 kg of fat. More importantly, during that time, she also gained muscle mass and bone density. Nothing about her approach was extreme. It was steady, structured, and realistic.

Around the same time, I started working with another client. He had consulted several well-known dietitians and followed multiple aggressive diet plans. Each time, he would lose about 8–10 kg in five to six months. The results were visible and motivating each time.

But once the diet ended, the structure disappeared. Eating became unregulated again, and the weight gradually came back, every single time.

He had been repeating this cycle for nearly four years by the time he came to me.

When you compare both starting points after several years, the contrast becomes very clear.

The woman, who focused on habits and consistency, was significantly lighter by 25 kg, stronger and healthier three years later.

The man, despite multiple 'successful' dieting phases over four years, was almost exactly where he had started.

The difference was not effort or intention.

It was sustainability.

Rapid weight loss often feels rewarding because the change is quick and visible. However, when progress is built on extreme restriction and tight control, it rarely becomes part of real life. And anything that cannot fit into daily life cannot be sustained.

When habits do not change, outcomes do not last.

Over time, it becomes clear that moderate, repeatable actions outperform extreme short-term efforts. Smaller changes, applied consistently, allow the body to adapt and allow the person to live.

That is how real transformation happens.

To Reiterate

- Food is not inherently good or bad. It is simply food. What matters is context, quantity, frequency, balance, beliefs, and your relationship with it.
- Awareness is the key to sustainable nutrition. Without it, portions feel restrictive and goals become stressful.
- Hunger timing can be used as feedback to understand whether a meal was balanced, not as a rule or judgement.
- Consistency is more important than intensity. Your body responds to patterns over time, not to specific days or one-off meals.
- The 80:20 approach introduces soulfulness, allowing room for enjoyment without guilt and reducing cycles of restriction and overeating.
- Sustainability is not forced; it emerges when awareness and soulfulness work together.

- Common diet mistakes often stem from extremes, moralising food, and ignoring hydration, balance or recovery.
- Use supplements as required.
- Extreme calorie deficits may lead to short-term results but often break sustainability and fuel the yo-yo cycle.
- The final habit is not restriction but reflection—using awareness to adjust gently instead of reacting harshly.
- Health is built through balance, flexibility and consistency, not perfection.

A Note from Me to You

This chapter is not about giving you rules to follow. It is meant to help you pause, reflect, and reconnect with what actually works in real life. If there is one thing I hope you take from this chapter, it is this: you do not need to do more; you need to do what already works, more consistently and with less fear.

From here on, let reflection guide you, not restriction. Adjust as life changes. Be gentle with your body. And remember, sustainability is not about control; it is about alignment. Food was never meant to be a battle.

It is meant to support life, health and well-being.

Habit 11

The habit of sustainability

The only habit I want to suggest now is actually not really a habit to add but a reminder to reflect.

Treat this chapter as a regular check-in, not a strict set of rules.

Whenever you feel stuck, frustrated, or tempted to go to extremes, ask yourself:

- Am I eating enough to support my energy levels, recovery and daily life?
- Are my portions aligned with my current goals and activity levels?

- Is my protein intake adequate across my meals?
- Am I eating enough fibre, vegetables and volume?
- Am I drinking enough water for my protein, fibre and supplement intake?
- Have I made space for enjoyment without feeling guilty?
- Does my current approach seem supportive or restrictive?
- Can I realistically keep this up for the next few months?

If something feels hard to sustain, do not push harder.
Adjust.
Reflection helps you to course-correct before burnout sets in.
Restriction breeds rebellion.
Reflection leads to regulation.
When you reflect:

- You stay connected to your body
- You catch the imbalance early
- You avoid extreme swings
- You maintain trust with food and with yourself

This is how awareness and soulfulness unite to foster sustainability.
You do not need to eat perfectly.
You should eat consistently, mindfully, and without fear.
Trust the process. You now have everything you need.

12

Movement and Strength: Use It or Lose It

MOVEMENT AND STRENGTH ARE the second pillar of health.

Most people do not realise that if food is the raw material, movement is the instruction manual.

Food supplies energy and building blocks, but it is movement, especially strength training, that directs the body where that energy should go. Without movement, the body's default system is storage. With movement, particularly resistance training, nutrients are sent to muscle repair, glycogen storage, stronger bones and improved metabolic function.

In simple terms, you do not just eat for health; you also move to determine how that food is used: either as fuel or as storage.

The body adapts to the signals it receives, not the intentions behind them.

And the body responds to that decision in a very predictable way. As discussed in earlier chapters, your actions continuously inform the body what to do, including what to eat. That is why it is important to understand the outcome of your actions.

There is a saying in the fitness industry: 'Use it or lose it.'

Nothing explains ageing and the human body better.

Ageing and Its Effects on the Human Body

As we age, some degree of physical loss is unavoidable. Muscle tissue, bone density, cartilage health, and overall structural strength gradually decline.

Up to about twenty years of age, the body is in a phase of growth and development. Around twenty to twenty-five years of age, growth plates close, and physical growth ceases. From the early twenties to around the forties, the body is generally at its strongest, most resilient, and best at recovering.

After thirty, the natural trend begins to shift towards a gradual decline.[1] Health markers may begin to change, muscle tone may decrease, recovery may slow, and tissues may become more vulnerable.

Ageing is inevitable. Rapid decline is not.

However, this decline happens at different rates for everyone.

What determines how quickly or slowly this deterioration occurs is stimulation or, in other words, physical activity.

Stimulation: The Deciding Factor

If you do not use what your body has, you will lose it faster.

That is the real meaning of 'use it or lose it'.

Loss happens naturally with age, but lack of movement accelerates it.

Movement does not prevent ageing, but it protects the body from rapid decline and unnecessary loss of muscle and connective tissue.

The human body thrives on stimulation.

- When you move, muscles retain tone and strength.
- When you exercise, the body adapts and becomes stronger.
- When you strength train, the body becomes even more resilient.

Your actions and how much you do largely determine the rate and extent of physical decline your body will experience over time.

The Two Parts of Movement

Movement can broadly be divided into two main categories.

Non-Exercise Activity Thermogenesis (NEAT)

This is the simplest and often overlooked type of movement.

> **Daily movement slows decline, even when formal exercise is absent.**

It includes everything that is not structured exercise, such as:

- Walking
- Sitting and standing
- Changing postures
- Daily chores
- Cooking
- Fidgeting
- General physical activity throughout the day

These are not structured workouts; they are ways of living an active life.

Even these unstructured movements help prevent complete physical stagnation[2], support baseline metabolic health, and slow down muscle loss. In simple terms, something is always better than nothing.

Focused, Structured Exercise

Structured exercise involves purposeful movement aimed at enhancing particular fitness elements. It can be divided into three components.

Strength Training

Everything 'uses' the body. Strength training 'builds' the body.

Everything you do 'uses' your body, but strength training 'builds' the body.

Strength training involves exerting resistance on muscles so they must contract, adapt and become stronger over time. During training, muscles develop small micro-tears. With adequate nutrition and rest, the body repairs these fibres, making them slightly stronger and more resilient.

This process maintains and improves muscle mass, strength and structural integrity.

Strength helps the body handle everyday life with less pain, improved posture, and a lower risk of injury. It is not restricted by age, gender or fitness level, and can be tailored to beginners, seniors, athletes and those recovering from injuries.

Strength training does not require extreme or maximal lifts to be effective. Muscle grows through consistent stimulation and progressive overload. Progression can occur through many variables, not just heavier weights, but also repetitions, tempo, range of motion and training frequency.

Strength training includes the following:

- Resistance training
- Bodyweight loading
- External load (machines, free weights, bands)

Strength is maintained only when the stimulus can progress.

The purpose of strength training is to:

- Preserve lean mass
- Improve bone density
- Support joints and connective tissue
- Improve glucose disposal
- Maintain resting metabolic rate

After the age of thirty-five to forty, strength training becomes essential; it is 'protective'.[3]

Flexibility

Training creates stress. Recovery teaches the body to come back to balance.

Flexibility is the ability to move joints and lengthen muscles.

On its own, flexibility is often overemphasised. When strength training with a full, controlled range of motion, separate flexibility exercises might not always be needed.

However, flexibility is essential after training. Stretching helps lengthen shortened muscles and signals the body to shift out of a stressed state. Exercise activates the sympathetic nervous system (fight-or-flight), while stretching and breathing help activate the parasympathetic nervous system (rest-and-digest), aiding recovery.

The body constantly balances between these two systems. Flexibility exercises help restore that balance. Practices like

Surya Namaskar followed by calm stretching and breathing illustrate this shift effectively.

Cardio Training

Cardio training focuses on the cardiovascular system: how efficiently the heart and lungs function.

Activities such as brisk walking, cycling, jogging or swimming are examples of aerobic training, in which the heart rate remains moderately elevated and can be maintained for longer durations.

Anaerobic training, on the other hand, involves short bursts of very high intensity followed by recovery periods, such as interval training or sprints.

Both forms strengthen the heart and lungs. When the cardiovascular system functions efficiently, blood circulation improves, nutrient delivery increases, and overall energy levels rise.

A stronger heart and lungs improve how the entire body functions.

Cardio activities that involve impact[4], such as jumping, skipping, jogging and running, offer an added benefit by stimulating bones to adapt and become denser.

Why Strength Matters More Than Most People Think

Being thin does not necessarily mean being fit, and muscle loss is not healthy weight loss. Muscle serves as a protector. It is a metabolic organ, not just for decoration.

Being thin is not the same as being strong.

- Muscles act as a glucose sink[5]
- They support insulin sensitivity
- They protect joints and the spine
- They improve hormonal signalling (including thyroid and reproductive hormones)
- They support ageing, independence and cognition

Sarcopenia, the loss of muscle mass, can start as early as the age of thirty in untrained individuals.

The Underrated Benefit of Exercise: Resilience

A Defining Challenge of Modern Life

Burnout has become a defining challenge of modern life. Constant demands—work pressure, family responsibilities, emotional burdens, poor sleep and lack of recovery—leave many people feeling drained, overwhelmed and out of touch with their bodies.

Burnout is not just mental; it also shows up physically as fatigue, poor recovery, low motivation, reduced strength, disturbed sleep and declining health markers. Rest alone often is not enough, because resilience is not rebuilt by avoidance; it is rebuilt through capacity. This is where movement and strength training play an underrated but critical role.

An Analogy: Resilience[6]

Built, not found

Resilience is the body's capacity to tolerate stress and recover from it: physically, mentally and emotionally.

Exercise trains this system.

Think of life as a long road filled with bumps, uneven surfaces, and occasional potholes. These represent stress: deadlines, illness, emotional strain and uncertainty. You cannot remove the road conditions; they are inevitable.

You can adjust your vehicle's suspension.

A weak, deconditioned body that is unused to stress feels every bump more sharply. Each pothole causes damage, fatigue and breakdown. Recovery takes longer and, eventually, the system struggles to keep going.

A body trained through regular movement and strength work develops stronger suspension. The bumps do not disappear, but they cause less disruption. The system absorbs stress better, stays stable and recovers faster.

Exercise does not reduce stress.

It increases your capacity to handle it.

Strength training, in particular, teaches the body to adapt under controlled stress. That adaptation translates into everyday life with better energy regulation, improved recovery, increased confidence, and a stronger sense of physical and mental steadiness.

Resilience, in this context, is not the same as toughness.

It is readiness.

And movement is one of the most reliable ways to build it.

Exercise Versus Nutrition: Understanding the Relationship

Many people believe that nutrition is the most important factor in body composition and health. Nutrition matters, but exercise determines how nutrition is utilised.

When you strength train and build muscle:

- Carbohydrates are directed towards muscles and stored as glycogen.
- Proteins are used to repair and rebuild muscle tissue that experiences micro-tears during training.
- Muscle growth and repair are stimulated.

An Analogy: Same Body, Different Signals

Imagine two men of the same age, height and weight. They eat similar foods and lead similar lives. On paper, they weigh the same. But their bodies look and function very differently.

Person A: Does not exercise

He does little to no structured movement and does not do strength training.

Over time, his body loses muscle and gains more fat, even though the scale stays the same. Muscles, not being regularly used, slowly shrink. Fat tissue gradually increases to store unused energy.

His calorie needs are lower because muscle is a more metabolically active tissue. With less muscle, his body needs fewer calories to sustain itself.

So, when he eats:

- Carbohydrates are less likely to be pulled into the muscle.
- Excess energy is more easily stored as fat.
- Protein has fewer active tissues to repair or build.

His body's message is straightforward: 'There is no regular demand for strength or muscle. Store energy for later.'

Person B: Exercises, including weight training

He moves regularly and weight trains regularly.

Even at the same body weight, he has more muscle and less fat, which makes him look leaner and more toned. His muscles are always being used, challenged and repaired.

The same food can send different signals and produce different outcomes.

Because muscle is metabolically active, his calorie needs are higher, even at the same body weight.

So, when he eats:

- Carbohydrates are directed towards muscles and stored as glycogen.

- Proteins are used to repair and rebuild muscle tissue.
- Less energy is pushed towards fat storage.

His body receives a very different message: 'Strength and muscle are required. Use incoming energy to support them.'

This improves insulin sensitivity, meaning carbohydrates are processed more efficiently, and proteins are utilised where they are needed most. This process is called nutrient partitioning[7], where nutrients are directed towards productive tissues, like muscle, instead of being stored as fat.

The scale tells you what you weigh. Movement determines what that weight is made of.

The Takeaway

The scale might show the same number, but the body composition and how food is used are completely different.

Food provides the raw material.

Exercise decides how that raw material is used.

Food provides material. Movement provides instruction.

A person who does not exercise is more likely to store excess energy as body fat. A person who exercises, especially with strength training, directs calories towards maintaining and building muscle.

This is especially relevant today, as conditions like diabetes are becoming increasingly common. The problem is often misunderstood. At a physiological level, the issue is usually insufficient muscle mass and decreased muscle activity, not just sugar or fat.

Muscle is one of the main tissues that take up glucose. When muscle mass is low or rarely stimulated, the body's ability to process carbohydrates decreases, leading to insulin resistance over time.

The problem is often not excess fat or sugar but insufficient muscle.

Strength training not only changes your appearance but also improves blood sugar control and metabolic health.

Why Movement Is a Core Pillar of Health

Together, strength training, flexibility and cardio support:

Use your body. Or lose it faster.

- Muscle preservation
- Bone health
- Joint integrity
- Metabolic efficiency
- Cardiovascular health
- Better circulation and nutrient delivery

The more you stay active, the slower your physical deterioration with age becomes.

Movement does not halt ageing.

But a lack of movement speeds up decline.

This is why movement and strength are essential, not optional. They are critical for long-term health, independence and quality of life.

Myths and Truths

1. *Myth:* 'If I eat well, exercise is optional.'

   Truth: Nutrition provides the raw material, but movement guides the body on how to use it. Without movement, especially strength training, the body is more likely to store energy rather than build or maintain muscle.

2. *Myth:* 'Walking is enough to maintain muscle as we age.'
   Truth: Walking is excellent for circulation and metabolic health, but it does not give enough stimulus to maintain muscle and bone mass over time. Strength training is necessary to slow down age-related muscle loss.
3. *Myth:* 'Strength training is only for athletes or young people.'
   Truth: Strength training is especially beneficial for adults over thirty-five to forty years of age. It helps preserve muscle mass, support joints, improve bone density and maintain independence as we age.
4. *Myth:* 'Thin people do not need to exercise.'
   Truth: Thinness does not necessarily mean having muscle mass, strength, or good metabolic health. It is possible to be thin yet metabolically unhealthy if muscle mass is low. Therefore, it is important for thin people to also focus on strength training.
5. *Myth:* 'Diabetes is only about sugar intake.'
   Truth: Muscle plays a major role in glucose disposal. Low muscle mass and activity decrease the body's ability to process carbohydrates, which can contribute to insulin resistance over time.
6. *Myth:* 'Weight training makes women bulky.'
   Truth: In reality, women need weight training even more than men. Women start with lower muscle mass and thinner bones, making strength training essential for muscle and bone health. Lifting weights does not make women bulky; building large muscle size requires years of specific training and a caloric surplus that most women never pursue.

To Reiterate

- Movement tells the body how to use food: either as fuel or as storage.
- Ageing is inevitable; rapid physical decline is not.
- What you stimulate, the body keeps. What you neglect, it lets go.
- Strength training does not just change how you look; it changes how your body functions.
- Muscle is not decoration; it is metabolic, structural and protective.
- Being thin is not the same as being strong or metabolically healthy.
- The same food can produce different outcomes, depending on the signal the body receives.
- Movement does not stop ageing, but lack of movement accelerates it.
- Use your body, or lose it faster.

A Note from Me to You

This chapter is not about forcing workouts or pushing yourself to exhaustion. It is about understanding how movement profoundly influences what your body becomes over time. Strength is not just about lifting the heaviest weights in the gym; it is about maintaining your ability to live well, move freely, recover better, and stay independent as you age. You do not have to do everything, but doing nothing always costs something.

If this chapter helps you see movement not as punishment or obligation, but as a biological requirement, then it has accomplished its goal. Understanding this is often more impactful than doing more. One simple way to apply this is a short, easy walk after meals, which can help muscles absorb glucose more efficiently, not by burning calories but by improving how food is processed.

13

Sleep, Stress, Recovery: Guard Your Sleep

GOOD QUALITY SLEEP IS essential for health and is often underrated. It is the third essential pillar of well-being, alongside nutrition and physical activity.

Sleep is not merely rest; it serves as a biological repair window that allows the body to recover, regulate, and adapt.

While sleep is important at every age, younger individuals generally find it easier to sleep well. However, as we age, both sleep quality and sleep duration decline. This decline is especially noticeable in women over forty, due to hormonal changes, increased stress, and slower recovery times, all of which can significantly impact sleep. At this stage in life, metabolism and overall health become far more sensitive to both sleep and stress.

Sleep is not an optional support; it is a foundation.

Key Functions of Sleep

During sleep, the body performs essential functions that are not as effective during waking hours. These functions include:

> **Sleep is not rest; it is repair.**

- Repair of muscles, joints, and connective tissue
- Regulation of metabolic and reproductive hormones
- Down-regulation of the nervous system and processing of emotions
- Maintenance of the immune system
- Repair of blood vessels and release of growth hormone
- Regulation of insulin response and appetite hormones

Sleep is not passive.

It is an active and restorative process that prepares the body for the demands of the following day.

How Much Sleep Is Enough?

Sleep needs are individual, not fixed.

The popular 'eight-hour' sleep rule is merely a guideline, not a biological law or a magic number.

For most adults, seven to nine hours of sleep is considered a healthy range. Research indicates that around seven hours of sleep is linked to the lowest health risks.

Some individuals function well on slightly less sleep, while others need more. Factors such as genetics, lifestyle, stress, training load, and life stage all impact sleep needs. What consistently poses a risk to health is chronic sleep deprivation, especially regularly getting less than six hours of sleep.[1]

Sleep Quality Matters

Sleep works best when it is enough, regular, and supported.

Using screens late at night can delay melatonin production, elevate stress hormones, and keep the brain alert long after the devices are put away. In contrast, exposure to natural daylight during the day supports the circadian rhythm and improves sleep quality at night.

There is no perfect number; consistency matters more than precision.

It is normal to take 10–30 minutes to fall asleep. If your mind feels restless, calming imagery or gentle music can help signal safety to your nervous system.

Risks of Insufficient Sleep

Consistently getting short or irregular sleep signals stress to the body. Over time, this can result in the following:

- Increased stress hormone activity
- Slower recovery and adaptation
- Reduced resilience to physical and emotional demands

Many people wake up at the same time each day due to their internal body clock, even after sleeping late. In such cases, avoiding late nights and establishing an earlier bedtime routine becomes especially important.

Active individuals often wake up early to exercise, even after sleeping late. While movement is beneficial, repeating this pattern over time can accumulate into chronic stress, which quietly affects health and performance.

Chronic sleep loss harms health more than occasional short nights.

How Sleep Affects Recovery

Recovery is not a state of inactivity; it is the body's ability to adapt.

Sleep is the foundation of this process. Without adequate sleep, muscle repair slows down, joint stiffness increases, and it becomes harder to recover from training stress. What may feel like 'lack of motivation' is often just unresolved fatigue.

Sleep quality supports recovery, metabolism, and mood.

How Sleep Affects Appetite and Metabolism

Poor sleep disrupts hormones that regulate appetite, leading to increased hunger and cravings the following day. This makes it harder to manage food intake, often resulting in overeating without awareness.

Slower fat loss is often a result of a sleep issue, not a matter of discipline.

How Sleep Affects Mood and Emotional Regulation

Sleep deprivation reduces emotional resilience. Irritability, low patience, anxiety, and mental fog are common signs of an under-rested nervous system. As sleep quality improves, mood stability and mental clarity often follow suit.

Gentle Reminder, Not a Rule

This is not just about perfection.

What matters more than achieving a perfect score is showing improvement over time. If your sleep is not ideal right now, try not to stress about it; stress disrupts sleep and recovery.

Stress disrupts sleep; compassion restores it.

Focus on gradually improving sleep habits by creating better conditions for rest and allowing for flexibility. Sleep, like nutrition, works best when approached with consistency and compassion rather than pressure.

Your nighttime routine directly impacts your health the following day.

Protect it with mindfulness rather than stress.

While nutrition fuels the body, sleep enables the body to effectively use that fuel. Without adequate rest, even the best nutrition plan will struggle to yield positive results.

Analogy: Sleep as Credit and Debt

Sleep functions like a credit system

Occasionally, you can borrow from your sleep reserves—whether due to late nights, travel, deadlines or family obligations. The body is adaptable enough to handle short periods of reduced sleep.

However, when sleep deprivation becomes frequent, it turns into a form of debt. Just like financial debt, the repercussions of sleep loss do not manifest immediately. The effects appear gradually and can include increased hunger and cravings, low patience, poor recovery, joint stiffness, slower fat loss and emotional instability.

The challenge is that willpower can temporarily mask the issue. Caffeine, sugar, motivation and discipline may help keep you functioning for a while, but they do not repay the debt. They merely postpone the inevitable consequences.

Sleep credit is accumulated through enough, regular, and restorative nights of rest. This credit increases your resilience, making it easier to train, work, and manage stress with greater ease.

Sleep debt, on the other hand, reduces your margin for error. Small stressors can feel bigger. Recovery takes longer. The same routine may become more difficult.

This is not about perfection. It is about having awareness.

Aim to consistently build your sleep credit and only borrow occasionally.

That is how sleep supports long-term health and recovery.

How the Pillars Work Together

- Nutrition: fuels the body
- Movement: signals adaptation
- Sleep: allows repair and regulation

Health is a system, not silos.

If one pillar is weak, the others need to work harder. When all three are supported, health becomes sustainable instead of effortful.

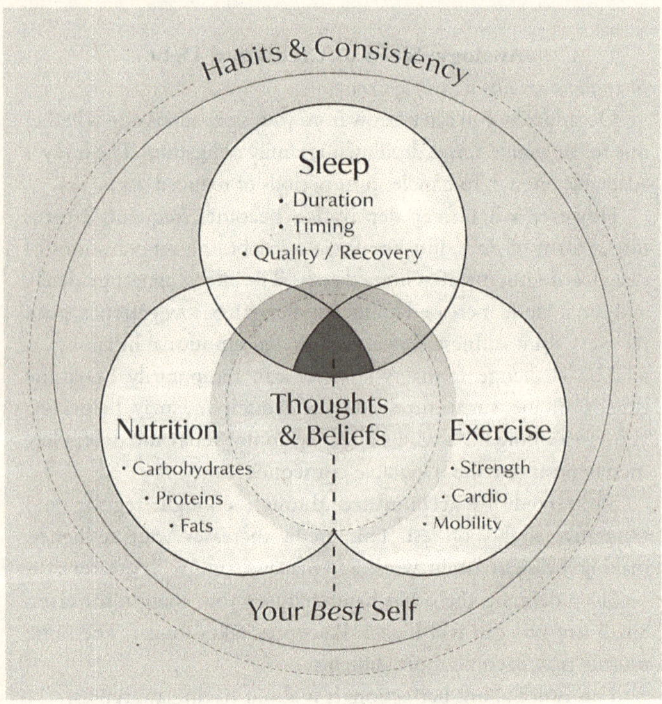

Figure 13.1: *The 'Fearless You' health system*

Myths and Truths

1. *Myth:* 'I can catch up on sleep over the weekend.'
   Truth: While occasional recovery sleep can help, chronic sleep debt cannot be fully repaid over the weekend. Irregular sleep patterns continue to strain hormones, recovery and metabolism.
2. *Myth:* 'If I am tired, I just need more motivation.'
   Truth: Persistent fatigue often stems from unresolved sleep debt, rather than a lack of discipline. Recovery is essential before motivation can follow.
3. *Myth:* 'More sleep is always better.'
   Truth: There is no universal sleep duration; consistency, quality, and alignment with one's lifestyle are more important than simply pursuing longer sleep.
4. *Myth:* 'Exercise can undo the damage of sleep deprivation.'
   Truth: Exercise supports health, but it cannot compensate for chronic sleep deprivation. Training signals adaptation, while sleep is the phase where adaptation actually occurs. Without adequate sleep, the stress from exercise accumulates rather than dissipates.
5. *Myth:* 'Train hard, regardless of the sleep.'
   Truth: Training effectiveness depends on recovery status. On days with poor sleep, lowering intensity or volume supports long-term progress more effectively than pushing through intense sessions.

To Reiterate

- Sleep is a foundational pillar of health, alongside nutrition and exercise.
- It is an active biological process that is essential for repair, recovery, hormonal regulation and emotional resilience.
- Sleep quality and needs change with age, stress levels, and hormonal shifts, especially in women over forty.

- The 'eight-hour rule' is merely a guideline, not a biological law; most adults function best within a seven- to nine-hour range.
- Chronic sleep deprivation, particularly when getting less than six hours of sleep, can consistently harm health and recovery.
- Poor sleep negatively impacts appetite regulation, metabolism, mood and training adaptation.
- Late nights combined with early mornings can gradually lead to chronic stress.
- Sustainable health is achieved by progressively improving sleep habits rather than striving for perfection.

A Note from Me to You

You do not need perfect sleep to be healthy; you just need enough rest, along with a willingness to improve gradually. Sleep is not something you control forcefully; it responds best to a sense of safety, rhythm and consistency. If your sleep is not ideal right now, try not to judge it harshly. Worrying about your sleep often makes the situation worse.

Instead, focus on creating better conditions for sleep. Protect your evenings whenever possible, and value recovery as much as you value effort. Similar to nutrition, sleep works best when approached with awareness, flexibility, and compassion.

14

Sample Diets: An Indian Context

Sample Diet 1: Vegan

Purpose

A fully plant-based diet can still meet protein, fibre, and micronutrient needs when planned with awareness.

Breakfast

- Fruit (seasonal)
- Soy milk/soy yoghurt
- *Poha*/oats *upma*/millet *upma* (made with vegetables and peas)

Lunch

- Salad (raw or lightly sauteed)
- *Dal*/*chana*/*rajma* (any one or mixed)
- Vegetable *sabzi* (seasonal, including leafy vegetables)
- Rice or *roti* (any grain or millet as per season)

Dinner

- Stir-fried or steamed vegetables
- Tofu/soy chunks/*dal*
- *Roti* or rice

Or

- *Dal*-rice-vegetable *khichdi*

Snack

- Sprouts salad/soya/*chana tikki*/edamame
- Roasted *chana*/peanuts/nuts and seeds
- Fruit or coconut water

Note: Four meals help distribute protein intake and energy more evenly throughout the day. Legumes and soy serve as the main protein sources, grains provide energy, salads add volume, fruits offer quick energy, and vegetables add variety and micronutrients. Rotate protein sources like *dal*s, beans, tofu, and soya. Include nuts and seeds for healthy fats and minerals. A plant-based protein supplement can be considered around workouts or when a meal lacks a clear protein source. Use other supplements as required. Tea or coffee, if desired, can be taken after any meal or snack.

Sample Diet 2: Vegetarian

Breakfast

- Fruit (seasonal)
- Low-fat milk/yoghurt
- *Paneer* stuffed *roti*/*poha*/oats *upma*/millet *upma* (made with vegetables and peas)

Lunch

- Salad (raw or lightly sauteed)
- *Paneer*/ *dal*/*chana*/*rajma* (any one or mixed)
- Vegetable *sabzi* (seasonal, including leafy vegetables)
- Rice or *roti* (any grain or millet as per season)
- Low-fat yoghurt (can give additional protein support)

Dinner

- Stir-fried or steamed vegetables
- Tofu/soy chunks/*paneer sabzi*/*dal*
- *Roti* or rice

Or

- *Dal*-rice-vegetable *khichdi* with yoghurt

Snack

- Buttermilk/yoghurt/sprouts salad/soya/*chana tikki*
- Roasted *chana*/peanuts/nuts and seeds
- Fruit or coconut water

Note: Four meals help distribute protein intake and energy more evenly throughout the day. Dairy foods such as milk, *paneer*, and yoghurt provide protein, along with legumes and *dals*. Grains provide fuel, salads add volume, fruits offer quick energy, and vegetables contribute variety and micronutrients. Rotate protein sources between dairy, *dals*, beans, and soy to prevent over-reliance on any single food. Nuts and seeds add healthy fats and minerals. A protein supplement may be considered around workouts or when meals lack a clear protein source. Use other supplements as required. Tea or coffee, if desired, can be taken after any meal or snack.

Sample Diet 3: Eggetarian

Breakfast

- Fruit (seasonal)
- Boiled egg/omelette/fried egg
- Milk/yoghurt

Lunch

- Salad (raw or lightly sauteed)
- Egg curry/*dal*/*chana*/*rajma* (any one or mixed)
- Vegetable *sabzi* (seasonal, including leafy vegetables)
- Rice or *roti* (any grain or millet as per season)
- Low-fat yoghurt (can give additional protein support)

Dinner

- Stir-fried or steamed vegetables
- Tofu/soy chunks/*dal*/boiled egg/omelette
- *Roti* or rice

Or

- *Dal*-rice-vegetable *khichdi*

Snack

- Eggs/buttermilk/yoghurt/sprouts salad/soya/*chana tikki*
- Roasted *chana*/peanuts/nuts and seeds
- Fruit or coconut water

Note: Four meals help distribute protein intake and energy more evenly throughout the day. Eggs are a high-quality protein source and can be combined with dairy and plant sources such as curd, *dal*s, and legumes. Grains provide fuel, salads add volume, fruits offer quick energy, and vegetables support micronutrient intake and dietary variety. Rotate protein sources among eggs, dairy, and plant proteins to maintain balance and digestive comfort. Include nuts and seeds for healthy fats and minerals. A protein supplement may be considered around workouts or when meals lack a clear protein source. Use other supplements only if required. Tea or coffee, if desired, can be taken after any meal or snack.

Sample Diet 4: Non-vegetarian

Breakfast

- Fruit (seasonal)
- Boiled egg/omelette/fried egg
- Milk/yoghurt

Lunch

- Salad (raw or lightly sauteed)
- Chicken/fish/egg curry/*dal*/*chana*/*rajma*
- Vegetable *sabzi* (seasonal, including leafy vegetables)
- Rice or *roti* (any grain or millet as per season)
- Low-fat yoghurt (can give additional protein support)

Dinner

- Stir-fried or steamed vegetables
- Tofu/soy chunks/*dal*/boiled egg/omelette/chicken/fish
- *Roti* or rice

Or
- *Dal*-rice-vegetable *khichdi*
- Chicken/fish salad

Snack
- Chicken/fish *tikka*
- Eggs/buttermilk/yoghurt/sprouts salad/soya/*chana tikki*
- Roasted *chana*/peanuts/nuts and seeds
- Fruit or coconut water

Note: Four meals help distribute protein intake and energy more evenly throughout the day. Animal foods such as poultry, fish, meat, and eggs act as primary sources of protein, supported by plant proteins from *dal*s and legumes. Grains provide fuel, salads add volume, fruits offer quick energy, and vegetables contribute fibre, micronutrients, and diversity. Rotate protein sources between animal and plant options rather than relying on a single type. Be mindful of visible and invisible fats from animal foods, and balance meals with vegetables. A protein supplement may be considered around workouts or when meals lack a clear protein source. Use other supplements only if necessary. Tea or coffee, if desired, can be taken after any meal or snack.

***Sample Diet 5: PG/Hostel Student** (Mess-based, Minimal Cooking)*

Purpose
To show how nutrition principles can still work with limited control, time, money and access to cooking.

Breakfast (Mess or outside)
- Fruit (if available)
- *Poha*/*upma*/*paratha*/bread slice(s) with butter
- Milk/yoghurt

Or
- Fruit (if available)
- *Idli/dosa* with *sambar*
- Milk/yoghurt

Upgrade (if possible):
- Add one or two boiled eggs or an omelette

Lunch (Mess or outside)
- Vegetable *sabzi*
- Rice or *roti*
- Chicken/egg/*dal/chana/paneer* curry
- Yoghurt (if available)

Dinner (Mess)
- Vegetable *sabzi*
- Chicken/egg/*dal/chana/paneer* curry
- *Roti* or rice

Snack (Between Classes)
- Roasted *chana*/peanuts
- Banana or apple

OR
- *Samosa*/puff/sandwich occasionally, paired with yoghurt, tea, or coffee

The following can be kept in the room as a snack/meal option:
- Fruit (if available)
- Rolled or instant oats/muesli
- Milk/yoghurt

Late-night/Emergency options
- Milk and bread
- Fruit
- Peanut *chikki*/nuts/*chana*
- Boiled eggs (if possible)

Note: Mess food is usually high in carbs; *dal* and yoghurt help balance protein intake and support digestion. Snacks are meant to be practical, not perfect. Try to include at least one protein source with every meal and snack. When meals often lack protein, a protein supplement can be considered—especially around workouts or on busy days when food options are limited. Instead of regularly buying chips and colas, opt for options like bananas, apples or yoghurt when available. Investing in a small popcorn maker can also be helpful—popcorn made from raw, dried corn kernels makes a good late-night snack, as it is high in fibre and provides high volume for better satiety. If paired with a cup of milk, it becomes a good meal.

Key PG/Hostel Survival Principles

- You cannot control the menu; control combinations.
- Add protein wherever possible, including supplements when needed.
- Buy cucumbers, carrots or fruits separately if access allows.
- Eat enough during the day to reduce late-night hunger pangs.
- Consistency beats 'clean eating' attempts that create stress.

Templates., Not Targets

These sample days are not ideals to pursue, but realities to embrace. Nutrition succeeds when it adapts to life, rather than forcing life to conform to food rules.

15

Food Glossary: Your Indian Kitchen Companion

Primary Carbohydrate Sources	**Primary Protein Sources**	**Primary Fat Sources**
Rice (all varieties) Wheat flour (*atta*) Quinoa Broken wheat (*dalia*) Oats (all varieties) Semolina (*rava/suji*) Flattened rice (*poha*) Puffed rice (*murmura*) Millets (*jowar, bajra, ragi, foxtail*, etc.) Puffed millets (all) *Sattu* Tapioca (*sabudana*) Potato/sweet potato Corn/*makki* Bread/*pav*/buns Oat milk Rice milk *Makhana* Popcorn Dried fruits (dates, prunes, figs, raisins, apricots, etc.) Sugar, jaggery, honey	All *dals* (*toor, moong, masoor, urad*) *Chana* (whole and *dal*) *Rajma* Chickpeas Soybean/tofu Edamame *Paneer* Milk Curd/yoghurt Buttermilk (*chaas/lassi*) Eggs Fish Chicken Meat Whey/plant protein powders Lactose-free milk Soy milk Pea protein milk Gram flour (*besan*)	*Ghee* Butter Coconut oil Oils (olive, mustard, groundnut, sesame, rice bran, sunflower, soybean) Cream/*malai* Coconut Peanuts Nuts (all types) Seeds (all types) Avocado Animal fat (from meat, eggs, dairy) Almond milk Coconut milk Cashew milk Mayonnaise Cheese Margarine

Table 15.1: *Common Indian food sources categorised by their primary macronutrient*

How to Read and Use This Glossary

This glossary is intended to guide you, not restrict you.

It is normal for a single food to provide more than one macronutrient. What matters is the role it most often plays on your plate.

Foods here are classified by their main nutritional role in the Indian diet. Actual meals are made up of combinations, portions and preparation methods, not isolated nutrients.

Vegetables and Leafy Greens: Where Do They Fit?

Technically, vegetables and leafy greens are carbohydrates, but this does not mean they act like grains or sugars in the body.

Most vegetables primarily contribute to:

- Fibre
- Volume
- Micronutrients
- Water

They add bulk and balance to meals while being lower in calories, so they are not a concentrated source of energy.

Leafy greens, in particular, are low in calories and digestible carbohydrates. Their value lies in being a good source of non-heme iron and in supporting digestion, insulin sensitivity, gut health, and overall nutrient intake. They are best viewed as foundational foods, meant to be eaten generously alongside all macronutrients.

Classifying vegetables as carbohydrates simply reflects their botanical and nutritional makeup, not their effect on blood sugar or body weight.

One Food, Multiple Nutrients

Many foods naturally contain a mix of carbohydrates, proteins, and fats.

For example:

- Milk provides carbohydrates, protein and fat.
- Nuts and seeds provide fat, along with some protein and fibre.
- *Dals* provide protein and carbohydrates.
- *Paneer* and cheese provide protein and fat.
- Eggs provide protein and fat.

This is why foods are grouped by their dominant contribution, not because they contain only that nutrient.

A food being listed under protein does not mean it contains no fat or carbs.

A food being listed under fat does not mean it lacks protein.

A food being listed under carbohydrates does not mean it is nutritionally inferior.

Same Source, Different Role

Some foods share the same ingredient but serve different nutritional roles depending on processing, portion size, and typical use.

For example:

- Whole *chana*, *besan* and *sattu* all come from gram but are eaten differently.
- Milk, curd and cream originate from dairy but contribute differently.
- Rice and puffed rice come from the same grain but function differently on the plate.

Processing changes how a food is used, how much is eaten at a time and what it primarily contributes to a meal. This is why origin alone cannot determine classification.

How to Use This in Daily Eating

Think of the glossary as a guide, not a rulebook.

When building a meal:

- Choose a clear primary complex carbohydrate.
- Add a dependable protein anchor.
- Include fat for satiety and absorption.
- Fill generously with vegetables and leafy greens.

No single food needs to do everything. Balance comes from a combination, not by forcing one item to provide all nutrients at once.

Variety Is Often Misunderstood

It does not mean that if you eat eggs today, you must have *poha* or *upma* tomorrow. Variety means rotating foods within each group—different *dal*s, vegetables, fruits and grains over time—rather than changing the entire meal every day.

A Final Note

Nutrition is most effective when it mirrors how people actually eat, not just how foods are listed on paper.

This glossary aims to reduce confusion, not establish food hierarchies.

Use it to understand roles, adjust portions and create meals that promote energy, health and sustainability without fear or rigidity.

Acknowledgements

This book is shaped by four people whose lives and values have profoundly influenced me.

My mother's journey made me confront health, resilience and genetic realities early in life. Despite years of physical challenges, she carried herself with quiet strength, grace and unwavering positivity. She chose courage over complaint, and though she is no longer here, her spirit continues to guide my choices, my work and the person I have become.

My father-in-law lived with optimism and purpose, facing life with resilience and composure. His journey taught me that positivity alone is not enough—awareness and action are equally important. Losing him pushed me towards creating awareness around health, nutrition and exercise, not from fear but from responsibility.

I am proud to be my father's daughter, from whom I learned to be truly fearless: to face challenges head-on, to not shy away from those stronger than me, and to think critically in the face of uncertainty. He uplifted those around him while constantly pushing himself to rise to a higher standard. That fearlessness is a part of who I am today.

My mother-in-law taught me quiet resilience: to carry on with grace and a smile. She often said, 'If something needs to be done, it will have to be done, whether we do it smiling or complaining is a choice.' Through her, I learned to move forward with calmness and without complaint.

Together, they have shaped my values, my voice and my purpose. Their strength, kindness and spirit live on in the work I do every day.

Notes

1 Getting Started

1 Roozendaal, Benno, Bruce S. McEwen, and Sumantra Chattarji. 'Stress, Memory and the Amygdala'. *Nature Reviews Neuroscience* 10, no. 6 (2009): 423–433.

2 Lally, Phillipa, Cornelia H.M. van Jaarsveld, Henry W.W. Potts, and Jane Wardle. 'How Are Habits Formed: Modelling Habit Formation in the Real World'. *European Journal of Social Psychology* 40, no. 6 (2010): 998–1009.

3 The Basics of Good Nutrition

1 European Parliament and Council of the European Union. *Regulation (EC) No 1924/2006 on Nutrition and Health Claims Made on Foods. Official Journal of the European Union*, 20 December 2006.

4 Hydration: The Zero-Calorie Drink

1 Dennis, Elizabeth A., A. Dengo, K. Comber, D. Flack, S. Savla, S. Davy, and B.M. Davy. 'Water Consumption Increases Weight Loss During a Hypocaloric Diet Intervention in Middle-Aged and Older Adults'. *Obesity* 18, no. 2 (2010): 300–307.

5 Breakfast: The First Meal of the Day Matters

1 Sutton, Emily F., R. Brooke Beyl, Kristine S. Early, William T. Cefalu, Eric Ravussin, and Courtney M. Peterson. 'Early Time-Restricted Feeding Improves Insulin Sensitivity, Blood Pressure, and Oxidative Stress Even Without Weight Loss in Men with Prediabetes'. *Cell Metabolism* 27, no. 6 (2018): 1212–1221.

2 Stalder, Tobias, Clemens Kirschbaum, Brigitte M. Kudielka, Emma K. Adam, Jens C. Pruessner, Stefan Wüst, Samantha Dockray, Nina

Smyth, Phil Evans, Dirk H. Hellhammer, Robert Miller, Mark A. Wetherell, Sonia J. Lupien, and Angela Clow. 'Assessment of the Cortisol Awakening Response: Expert Consensus Guidelines'. *Psychoneuroendocrinology* 170 (2024): 106209.

3 Farshchi, H.R., M.A. Taylor, and I.A. Macdonald. 'Deleterious Effects of Omitting Breakfast on Insulin Sensitivity and Fasting Lipid Profiles in Healthy Lean Women'. *The American Journal of Clinical Nutrition* 81, no. 2 (2005): 388–396.

4 Astbury, Nerys M., Helen A. Taylor, and Richard D. Mattes. 'Consumption of Solid Food Compared with Breakfast Skipping Improves Appetite Control and Satiety Responses'. *Physiology & Behavior* 199 (2019): 168–173.

6 Balanced Meal Frequency

1 Teff, Karen L. 'Cephalic Phase Insulin Release in Humans: Mechanism and Function'. *Physiology & Behavior* 176 (2017): 11–17.

2 St-Onge, Marie-Pierre, Frank M. Phillips, and Shahrad Taheri. 'Meal Frequency and Timing: Impact on Metabolic Disease Risk'. *Current Opinion in Endocrinology, Diabetes and Obesity* 26, no. 5 (2019): 1–7.

3 Pot, Gerda K. 'Meal Irregularity and Cardiometabolic Consequences: Results from Observational and Intervention Studies'. *Proceedings of the Nutrition Society* 77, no. 4 (2018): 475–486.

4 Schoenfeld, Brad J., Alan A. Aragon, Eric T. Wilborn, Lem W. Krieger, and James W. Sonmez. 'Body Composition Changes Associated with Fasted Versus Non-Fasted Aerobic Exercise'. *Journal of the International Society of Sports Nutrition* 11, no. 54 (2014): 1–6.

7 Carbohydrates: Friends, Not Foes

1 Mergenthaler, Philipp, Uwe Lindauer, Gerald A. Dienel, and Andreas Meisel. 'Sugar for the Brain: The Role of Glucose in Physiological and Pathological Brain Function'. *Trends in Neurosciences* 36, no. 10 (2013): 587–597.

2 Makki, Kassem, Emmanuelle Deehan, Jan Walter, and Fredrik Bäckhed. 'The Impact of Dietary Fiber on Gut Microbiota in Host Health and Disease'. *Cell Host & Microbe* 23, no. 6 (2018): 705–715.

3 Chandalia, Manisha, Amit Garg, Dieter Lutjohann, Klaus von Bergmann, Scott M. Grundy, and Latha Jialal. 'Beneficial Effects of High Dietary Fiber Intake in Patients with Type 2 Diabetes Mellitus'. *The New England Journal of Medicine* 342, no. 19 (2000): 1392–1398.

4 DiMeglio, Daniel P., and Richard D. Mattes. 'Liquid versus Solid Carbohydrate: Effects on Food Intake and Body Weight'. *International Journal of Obesity* 24, no. 6 (2000): 794–800.

5 Reynolds, Andrew, Jim Mann, Nikki Cummings, Julie Winter, Lisa Mete, and Ailsa Wood. 'Carbohydrate Quality and Human Health: A Series of Systematic Reviews and Meta-Analyses'. *The Lancet* 393, no. 10170 (2019): 434–445.

6 World Health Organization. *Guideline: Sugars Intake for Adults and Children*. Geneva: World Health Organization, 2015.

7 National Institute of Nutrition. *Dietary Guidelines for Indians*. Hyderabad: National Institute of Nutrition, 2020.

8 Flood-Obbagy, Jennifer E., and Barbara J. Rolls. 'The Effect of Fruit in Different Forms on Energy Intake at a Meal'. *Appetite* 52, no. 2 (2009): 416–422.

9 Holloszy, John O. 'Regulation of Glucose Transport into Skeletal Muscle'. *Reviews of Physiology, Biochemistry and Pharmacology* 150 (2005): 1–30.

10 Salmerón, Jorge, Ascherio Alberto, Eric B. Rimm, Graham A. Colditz, Donna Spiegelman, Walter C. Willett, and Meir J. Stampfer. 'Dietary Fiber, Glycemic Load, and Risk of NIDDM in Men'. *Diabetes Care* 20, no. 4 (1997): 545–550.

8 Proteins: Your Body's Building Blocks

1 Cruz-Jentoft, Alfonso J., Gülistan Bahat, Jürgen Bauer, Yves Boirie, Olivier Bruyère, Tommy Cederholm, Cyrus Cooper, et al. 'Sarcopenia: Revised European Consensus on Definition and Diagnosis'. *Age and Ageing* 48, no. 1 (2019): 16–31.

2 Wolfe, Robert R. 'The Concept of Limiting Amino Acids in Dietary Protein and Its Role in Human Nutrition'. *Advances in Nutrition* 15, no. 3 (2024): 100186.

3 Food and Agriculture Organization of the United Nations and World Health Organization. *Protein Quality Evaluation in Human Nutrition: Report of an FAO Expert Consultation.* Rome: Food and Agriculture Organization of the United Nations, 2013.

4 Boirie, Yves, Michel Dangin, Patricia Gachon, Bernard Vasson, Jean-Louis Maubois, and Beaufrère Bernard. 'Slow and Fast Dietary Proteins Differently Modulate Postprandial Protein Accretion'. *Proceedings of the National Academy of Sciences of the United States of America* 94, no. 26 (1997): 14930–14935.

5 Wolfe, Robert R. 'The Underappreciated Role of Muscle in Health and Disease'. *The American Journal of Clinical Nutrition* 84, no. 3 (2006): 475–482.

6 Moore, Daniel R., Sarah M. Phillips, Jason E. Babraj, Kevin Smith, and Michael J. Rennie. 'Myofibrillar and Mitochondrial Protein Synthesis in Human Skeletal Muscle in Response to Ingested Protein Dose'. *The American Journal of Clinical Nutrition* 89, no. 1 (2009): 161–168.

7 Phillips, Stuart M. 'Physiologic and Molecular Bases of Muscle Hypertrophy and Atrophy: Impact of Resistance Exercise on Human Skeletal Muscle'. *The Journal of Applied Physiology* 103, no. 1 (2007): 345–353.

8 Areta, Jose L., David W. Burke, Lachlan M. Ross, David M. Camera, Justin M. West, Alan Garnham, David T. Moore, et al. 'Timing and Distribution of Protein Ingestion During Prolonged Recovery from Resistance Exercise Alters Myofibrillar Protein Synthesis'. *The Journal of Physiology* 591, no. 9 (2013): 2319–2331.

9 Greenhaff, Paul L., Daniel Karagounis, Stephanie Peirce, Mike Simpson, Philip Hazell, Andrew Layfield, Dan Wackerhage, et al. 'Disassociation between the Effects of Amino Acids and Insulin on Signalling, Ubiquitin Ligases, and Protein Turnover in Human Muscle'. *The Journal of Physiology* 586, no. 20 (2008): 4825–4835.

10 Westerterp, Klaas R. 'Diet Induced Thermogenesis'. *Nutrition & Metabolism* 1, no. 5 (2004): 1–5.

11 Jäger, Ralf, Chad M. Kerksick, Bill I. Campbell, Paul J. Cribb, Shawn D. Wells, Tim Ziegenfuss, Abbie E. Ferrando, et al. 'International Society of Sports Nutrition Position Stand: Protein and Exercise'. *Journal of the International Society of Sports Nutrition* 14, no. 20 (2017): 1–25.

12 Indian Council of Medical Research–National Institute of Nutrition. *Indian Food Composition Tables*. Hyderabad: National Institute of Nutrition, 2017.

13 Jäger, Ralf, Chad M. Kerksick, Bill I. Campbell, Paul J. Cribb, Shawn D. Wells, Tim Ziegenfuss, Abbie E. Smith-Ryan, and Jose Antonio. 'International Society of Sports Nutrition Position Stand: Protein and Exercise'. *Journal of the International Society of Sports Nutrition* 14, no. 20 (2017): 1–25.

9 Fats: Fats Do Not Make You Fat

1 Bazinet, Richard P., and Stephan Layé. 'Polyunsaturated Fatty Acids and Their Metabolites in Brain Function and Disease'. *Nature Reviews Neuroscience* 15, no. 12 (2014): 771–785.

2 Bazinet, Richard P., and Stephan Layé. 'Polyunsaturated Fatty Acids and Their Metabolites in Brain Function and Disease'. *Nature Reviews Neuroscience* 15, no. 12 (2014): 771–785.

3 Hooper, Lee, Jonathon Martin, Abigail Abdelhamid, and George Davey Smith. 'Reduction in Saturated Fat Intake for Cardiovascular Disease'. *Cochrane Database of Systematic Reviews* 5 (2020): CD011737.

4 Schwingshackl, Lukas, and Georg Hoffmann. 'Monounsaturated Fatty Acids and Risk of Cardiovascular Disease: A Systematic Review and Meta-Analysis'. *Annals of Nutrition and Metabolism* 63, no. 4 (2013): 314–324.

5 Marklund, Matti, Wu H. Sampson, Frank B. Hu, Dariush Mozaffarian, et al. 'Biomarkers of Dietary Omega-6 Fatty Acids and Incident Cardiovascular Disease: A Pooled Analysis of 30 Prospective Cohort Studies'. *Circulation* 141, no. 3 (2020): 242–253.

6 Fleming, Jennifer A., and Penny M. Kris-Etherton. 'Effect of Dietary Alpha-Linolenic Acid and Marine Omega-3 Fatty Acids on Cardiovascular Risk Factors'. *The American Journal of Clinical Nutrition* 89, no. 2 (2009): 618–624.
7 Medzhitov, Ruslan. 'Origin and Physiological Roles of Inflammation'. *Nature* 454, no. 7203 (2008): 428–435.
8 Simopoulos, Artemis P. 'The Importance of the Omega-6/ Omega-3 Fatty Acid Ratio in Cardiovascular Disease and Other Chronic Diseases'. *Experimental Biology and Medicine* 233, no. 6 (2008): 674–688.
9 de Souza, Russell J., Andrew Mente, Anna Maroleanu, Anita Cozma, Vanessa Ha, Teresa Kishibe, Ellen Uleryk, et al. 'Intake of Saturated and Trans Unsaturated Fatty Acids and Risk of All-Cause Mortality, Cardiovascular Disease, and Type 2 Diabetes: Systematic Review and Meta-Analysis of Observational Studies'. *BMJ* 351 (2015): h3978.
10 Grootveld, Martin, Christopher Silwood, and Kerry C. Grootveld. 'Chronic non-communicable disease risks presented by lipid oxidation products in fried foods'. *Foods* 11, no. 2 (2022): 1–18.
11 World Health Organization. *WHO Guidelines on Total Fat, Saturated Fat and Trans-Fat Intake for Adults and Children*. Geneva: World Health Organization, 2023.

12 Movement and Strength: Use It or Lose It

1 Janssen, Ian, Steven B. Heymsfield, Zhenming Wang, and Ross Roubenoff. 'Skeletal Muscle Mass and Distribution in 468 Men and Women Aged 18–88 yr'. *Journal of Applied Physiology* 89, no. 1 (2000): 81–88.
2 Levine, James A., Liane M. Eberhardt, and Michael D. Jensen. 'Role of Nonexercise Activity Thermogenesis in Resistance to Fat Gain in Humans'. *Science* 283, no. 5399 (1999): 212–214.
3 Westcott, Wayne L. 'Resistance Training Is Medicine: Effects of Strength Training on Health'. *Current Sports Medicine Reports* 11, no. 4 (2012): 209–216.
4 Watson, Scott L., Belinda S. Weeks, David J. Weis, Aaron L. Harding, and Belinda R. Beck. 'High-Intensity Resistance and

Impact Training Improves Bone Mineral Density and Physical Function in Postmenopausal Women with Low Bone Mass: The LIFTMOR Randomized Controlled Trial'. *Journal of Bone and Mineral Research* 33, no. 2 (2018): 211–220

5 DeFronzo, Ralph A., Ele Ferrannini, Leif Groop, Rury R. Holst, Xilin Hu, Philip M. Pratley, and Francesco Giorgino. 'Type 2 Diabetes Mellitus'. *Nature Reviews Disease Primers* 1 (2015): 15019

6 Stubbs, Brendon, Lee Smith, Joseph Firth, Simon Rosenbaum, Felipe Schuch, and Ai Koyanagi. 'Physical Activity and Fitness as Protective Factors Against Stress-Related Disorders: A Systematic Review'. *Journal of Affective Disorders* 294 (2021): 546–556.

7 Areta, Jose L., David Camera, Lachlan M. West, Justin M. Broad, Darren Burke, David R. Moore, David M. Phillips, et al. 'Timing and Distribution of Protein Ingestion During Prolonged Recovery from Resistance Exercise Alters Myofibrillar Protein Synthesis'. *The Journal of Physiology* 591, no. 9 (2013): 2319–2331.

13 Sleep, Stress, Recovery: Guard Your Sleep

1 Spiegel, Karine, Rachel Leproult, and Eve Van Cauter. 'Impact of Sleep Debt on Metabolic and Endocrine Function'. *The Lancet* 354, no. 9188 (1999): 1435–1439.

About the Author

Mitushi Ajmera is a wellness and movement coach driven by one belief: the body is always speaking to us, and we are always speaking back, through how we eat, move, rest and recover. Her own fitness journey began in extremes: rapid weight loss, overtraining, injury, healing and, finally, education. That breakdown became her breakthrough and shaped her path in the industry. For over fourteen years, she has worked as a senior master trainer, with international certifications in fitness and sports nutrition, functional and fitness training, Pilates and yoga. She has had the privilege of bringing wellness education to corporate platforms and universities, sharing ideas on the TEDx stage and in the media, and advocating a mindful, science-meets-intuition approach to training. Today, her work focuses on helping people move better, recover smarter, nourish themselves without fear and build strength from within, transforming not through restriction but through understanding.